Also by Barney J. Kenet, M.D.,
and Patricia Lawler

SAVING YOUR SKIN:
Prevention, Early Detection, and Treatment
of Melanoma and Other Skin Cancers

America's Leading Dermatologist Reveals the Essential Secrets for Youthful, Radiant Skin

Barney J. Kenet, M.D.

with Patricia Lawler

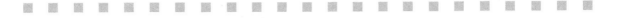

How to

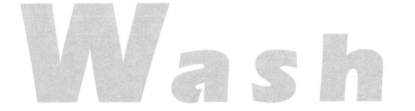

Your

Face

SIMON & SCHUSTER

SIMON & SCHUSTER
Rockefeller Center
1230 Avenue of the Americas
New York, NY 10020

Copyright © 1999 by Dr. Barney J. Kenet
and Patricia Lawler
All rights reserved, including the right of reproduction
in whole or in part in any form.
SIMON & SCHUSTER and colophon are registered trademarks
of Simon & Schuster Inc.
Anatomical drawings by Jackie Aher
Designed by Karolina Harris
Manufactured in the United States of America
10   9   8   7   6   5   4   3   2   1
Library of Congress Cataloging-in-Publication Data
Kenet, Barney J., date.
    How to wash your face : America's leading
dermatologist reveals the essential secrets for youthful,
radiant skin / Barney J. Kenet; with Patricia Lawler.
        p.   cm.
    1. Face—Care and hygiene.   2. Skin—Care and
hygiene.   I. Lawler, Patricia, date.   II. Title.
RL87.K46   1999
646.7'26—dc21   99-15528   CIP
ISBN 0-684-85282-9 (alk. paper)

The ideas, procedures and suggestions in this book are intended to supplement, not replace, the medical advice of the reader's own health care professional. All matters regarding your health require medical supervision. The reader should consult with a health care professional before adopting any of the advice in this book as well as about any condition that may require diagnosis or medical attention. The authors and the publisher expressly disclaim any responsibility for any liability, loss or risk, personal or otherwise, arising directly or indirectly from the use and application of any of the contents of this book.

    The medical anecdotes presented in this book are drawn from Dr. Kenet's experiences with patients. In order to protect the patients' privacy, names and identifying details have been changed and/or composites used whenever patients are discussed in this book.

Acknowledgments

We are blessed to have so many wonderful people around us. The love of our family remains a constant source of support. David Kenet, as father, physician and advisor, has given me the confidence to succeed and the inspiration to practice medicine with skill and compassion. He is the one who encouraged me to pursue a career in dermatology, and it has been one of the best decisions I have ever made.

Valerie Kenet's enthusiasm, support and pride in her children bring out the best in all of us.

Stacia Kenet Lansman, M.D., who in the midst of her busy life found the time to help us, deserves our gratitude and always has our love.

To our other wonderful family members: Robert Kenet, M.D., Steffi Seligman Kenet, Brian and Myrian Kenet, Monica and Tom Gold, Catherine and Justin Giovanetti, Ron Reeves, Anthony and Billy Lawler Jr., and Bill Sr. and Joey.

Thanks to special friends Tom Lavagnino, Hope Levy, Bettina Kamriani and Debbie Russo, and to our careful readers Fiona McConnell and Leigh Devine. For special help on issues relating to cosmetics and makeup, we would like to thank Mark Carasquillo and Maria Verel.

We also acknowledge the talent of Hester Kaplan, who helped to make this book clear and simple. Thank you to Arthur Rhodes, M.D., M.P.H., for your able assistance with the chapter on aging skin. I would also like to thank Philip G. Prioleau, M.D., a generous mentor and teacher.

Writing a book requires hours of solitude and concentration that would not have been possible without the dedication and loving care of Mia Poppick who managed to keep things quiet.

To the staff at New York Presbyterian Hospital/Cornell Medical Center Library for their assistance in research.

David Rosenthal, we thank you for ending the struggle to find the right title for this book and for taking this book with you in your travels.

The most artful editor's work goes unnoticed, almost by definition. Thus it is incumbent upon us to publicly thank Zoe Wolff for working with us to create a worthy finished product.

Our friend Laura Day has a generous heart and shared much with us. Our success had its beginnings with her support. Her loyalty is most rare.

Finally, to our agent Melanie Jackson, our thanks for her gracious manner and skillful attention to details great and small. Let's do another.

To Our Miss Lovely, Isabelle Catherine

Contents

I grew up in a family of physicians. My father, an ear, nose and throat surgeon, practiced for over twenty years in Lakeland, Florida, a small town
in the citrus belt. My older brother, Robert, a cardiologist, preferred big
cities and practices in New York. My sister, Stacia, a pediatrician, enjoys
the slower pace of country living and works in a clinic serving poor families in northern California. She has recently become interested in alternative medicine and has integrated those philosophies into her practice.

My training as a dermatologist began at New York Presbyterian Hos-
pital/Cornell Medical Center. There, I saw a broad range of problems—
from hospitalized patients with life-threatening blistering diseases to
clinic patients with acne and poison ivy. I am now in private practice in
New York City and see many people with cosmetic rather than medical
concerns. My family background as well as my formal education have
provided me with an appreciation for both the technical and human sides
of patient care.

Although cosmetic concerns make up the bulk of this book, you will
find important health information as well. In my first book, *Saving Your
Skin,* the message was clear: *Get to your doctor's office as soon as possible if you suspect you have skin cancer, particularly melanoma.*

Doing so could save your life. Here, the point is altogether different. Instead of telling you to run to the doctor's, I want you to stay away—from me and anyone else offering cosmetic services—for as long as possible. How can I help you do this? By teaching you how you can help yourself.

I will provide you with information about your skin profile, an analysis that goes beyond the overly simplistic skin types: dry, oily or combination. Anyone who is over twenty knows that his or her skin is more than a pool of over- or underactive oil glands. Our skin and our overall appearance are influenced by where we live, our hormones, stress, pregnancy, menopause, diet, alcohol consumption and smoking, to name a few factors. (And these can change from month to month.)

I will also teach you about old-fashioned home care. Many of the products I recommend are simple, inexpensive, over-the-counter goods. You may already own some but simply don't know how to use them to your best advantage. For those of you who are interested in alternative and herbal remedies for skin problems, I have devoted a chapter to those issues as well.

I wrote this book to teach you how to take better care of your skin and your health in general. I won't offer you tips on trends or fads like many women's magazines do—to the delight of their major advertiser, the cosmetic industry. My financial security does not depend on the endorsement of any of the products, techniques or professionals mentioned in this book. Rather, I depend on the satisfaction of my patients who trust my judgment *even when I tell them to delay the use of cosmetic surgery for the best results.*

I will show you how to improve your appearance, your vitality and your attitude. This book is about discovering what is best for you at your age, with your budget, with your skin type, your medical history and your emotional makeup.

Many of my patients are affluent, medically sophisticated New Yorkers—high achievers, perfectionists. I have also been flattered by patients who come from Argentina, Switzerland, Saudi Arabia and Italy to see me. I also see patients without much in the way of social or economic wealth. While their concerns and priorities may be a bit different from those of the Park Avenue executive and international traveler, their desire to look attractive and healthy is the same. Because they don't have quite as much money to spend, I make sure to find a way within their budget to get results.

People who want to look better are vulnerable. They feel old, tired and out of place in a society that venerates tight skin and big muscles over wisdom and grace. That is another reason I wrote this book: *I want to turn you into a discerning consumer of cosmetic care regardless of your age, education or income.*

Once you have made the decision to see a doctor about improving your appearance, I want you to walk into his or her office well prepared. This book will show you how to interview your doctor, ask the right questions and avoid unnecessary treatment. I will show you how to work with your doctor by developing a partnership.

I will explain what a physician can offer patients without using a scalpel.

I will show you how to choose an honest, ethical physician who will put your health and appearance ahead of his or her financial incentives. Sometimes doctors with the best intentions persuade their patients to undergo unneeded surgery. *You, the patient, must stay in control.*

In most situations a person sees a doctor to complain about a specific symptom. In the field of dermatology, things are a little different. Often my patients are vaguely unhappy about the way they look but don't know what they need or even what exactly is bothering them about their appearance. An extra crinkle around the eyes, dull skin, sometimes even an unexpected career change or a rocky marriage prompts some people to see me.

This book was written to help people define their expectations and realize their goals for healthier, better-looking skin. It provides a means for everyone to achieve an improved appearance. I hope you enjoy reading it.

Introduction

Patients come to me wanting to know more about their skin. It is a subject that can confuse even the most intelligent person because of the information and misinformation that barrages us every day.

My purpose in writing this book is to help you understand how your skin works, why it looks the way it does and what you can do to improve it, regardless of your age. There are a lot of books available by eminent skin specialists who claim they have the answer to looking young. It's tempting to think there is truly only one way to take care of all your skin problems. But the truth is, no single procedure, no one cream can do everything for everyone. Moreover, all the high-tech treatments and all the money in the world cannot replace what you must do for yourself every day at home. That's where it begins.

In order for you to be effective in caring for your skin, I have created a Skin Profile system. Instead of listing skin by "types," I use the phrase Skin Profile. I specifically chose the word "profile" because of its definition: "an analysis of the history and status of a process or relationship." To me, this is precisely how your skin should be viewed. Your personal Skin Profile is more than a category or type. It is really a process—a dynamic, fluid and ongoing event. How your skin looks depends on the inner workings of your body, your state of mind, your environment and your willingness to do all you can to improve these interdependent factors. Of course, heredity plays a big role as well, but you can work with the genes that nature gave you to maximize your personal best.

You will be learning whether your skin responds and reacts most strongly to internal forces or external ones. For example, Hormonally Reactive Skin responds to the chemical changes within your body that ebb and flow at various levels, day to day, month to month, year to year. Individuals with Stress-Reactive Skin notice that variable emotions change the appearance of their skin more than anything else.

Other readers will discover that the outside world leaves its mark on their skin. Persons with Environmentally Sensitive Skin experience irritation, rashes, breakouts and other problems when their skin comes in contact with perfumes, dyes and cosmetic ingredients, for example. I will show you how to eliminate irritants and allergens while maintaining a skin care regimen that will bring out the best in your skin. The environment can harm your skin over the long run as well. Too much sun and wind as well as other habits like smoking result in Overexposed Skin. Finally, I will briefly discuss how to keep Hearty Skin looking good. People with Hearty Skin look younger than people of the same age and find that using basic inexpensive products works well.

My approach to skin care has always been to ask my patients in-depth questions during each visit. Learning everything about a person makes caring for his or her skin easier. When you read this book, you will be treated like one of my patients. I will ask you many questions—not just about your skin but about who you are and how you live. Your answers will provide the information that determines how best to care for your skin.

At first you may wonder about the relevance of certain questions when it comes to treating your skin. However, you will soon see that all the answers have a bearing on you, your lifestyle, your health and, by definition, your skin.

With that analysis complete, your daily skin care routine will become much simpler. I am committed to saving you time, money and effort. I want to support you in your quest to look great without a doctor's help and without unneeded risk to your well-being.

You will find that I have recommended a number of specific brand-name products. My choices are dependent on my personal experience, patients' suggestions and a review of the ingredients in the product. More than one product is given in each category to give you an opportunity to purchase items at a drugstore for usually under $20 or at a department store for usually over $20. The order in which the product is listed does not indicate preference. I have made an effort to choose items from a variety of sources. I have also limited my list to widely available national brands made by companies that have a long history of standing behind their products.

This book covers all there is to know about skin care. It also helps you decide how to select a doctor (if you choose to see one) who suits your needs.

After you have finished this book, I am sure you will never think about your skin in the same way again. I am also sure that your skin will look and feel better. People will notice, but, more important, you will too.

How to Wash Your Face

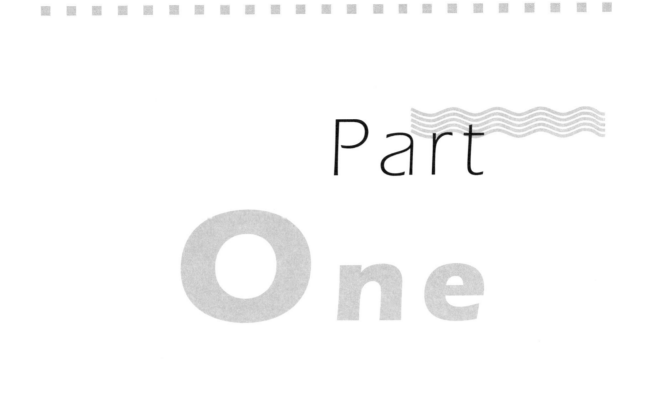

Part

One

1

The Path to Beauty

What price beauty? A $19,000 face-lift, a $200-per-hour personal trainer or a $3 pair of support hose?

How far will you go to look better? To the corner drugstore for a jar of cold cream or across the country for six-hour surgery under general anesthesia?

When do you start? At sixteen to carve a button nose or at thirty-five when crinkles become crow's feet or at sixty-five or later?

These questions resonate with particular significance for me because I see people every day who want to know what they can do for themselves, or with my help, to look their best. Some people will do "whatever it takes" to look as good as possible. They want the latest treatment, especially anything new they come across in a magazine. There are others who simply want to know how to keep their skin looking healthy and feeling soft and smooth.

In a single week at my office I come across people with itchy, raw skin, flaky scalps, red eyes, terrible sunburns, infected nails and cracked lips. Some patients require intense medical care, but most just need simple instructions about everyday skin care. Washing, shaving, moisturizing and even the mundane task of drying your skin have a significant impact on the way you look.

Many patients come to me after trying to help themselves. They have wasted money on expensive creams and lotions. They have aggravated their skin problems by using harsh products or have ignored other conditions that require attention. I often hear the same questions: "Why is my face so dry?" "I stay out of the sun, so why am I still getting brown spots?" "Should I be getting acne at my age?"

Even more basic than that, *some people don't even know how to wash their face.*

■ The Six Virtues of Successful Skin Care

If you have tried to care for your skin but are still not satisfied with the results, you need to learn why your skin is not responding, and to stop making the same mistakes over and over. You need to use skin products that protect and enhance instead of irritate and cover up problems. Most important, you need to gain insight into the way you see yourself.

You *can* look younger. Your skin *can* look smooth and radiant. Before you can expect to achieve these goals, however, you must learn the Six Virtues of Successful Skin Care. Follow them, and not only will your efforts lead to a better-looking you, but you will have fun in the process and even save money.

1. COMMITMENT
Know How Far You Will Go to Get the Results You Want

- Would you like to improve the appearance of your skin, hair or nails?
- Do you feel that you look older than your actual age? If so, how much does it bother you?
- Do you think about your skin and its appearance every day or once a week—or do you start to worry only when you have a problem?

- Are you willing to stick to a daily regimen and achieve gradual improvement over time, or do you want quick results?
- Are you willing to take time off from work to accomplish your goals?
- How much money can you spend to improve your appearance?
- Is your desire to improve your appearance based on the opinion of another person or a recent event in your life such as a divorce?
- Do you think you are doing everything possible to improve your appearance as part of a daily at-home skin care routine?
- Do you have fears about a cosmetic procedure that you have been considering?
- Have you found a doctor you can trust who is willing to take the time to help you?

The answers to these questions say a lot about you. They help identify your personal risk/benefit ratio. In other words, how much risk are you willing to accept for a particular cosmetic benefit? By "risk" I don't mean just potential medical complications, although those issues are very important. I mean all the expense, time and energy you are willing to expend to reach your goals.

As a physician I must take into account a person's health status and medical history before recommending any course of treatment. Only after all the medical issues have been explored can we come to a decision about what to do from a cosmetic point of view. The chapters that follow will provide you with essential information about your Skin Profile. This will be obtained by viewing in a systematic way how your personal habits, heredity and lifestyle influence the condition of your skin. You will discover reasons for the state of your skin that you probably never even considered and will learn what you can do to correct your problems.

Understanding your own habits and lifestyle is critical. I rarely give patients more than two skin care products to use at a time. Too much information, too many prescriptions and too much advice in one session overwhelms. I always take into account what the patient will and won't do to look better. Assuming that everyone has the same level of interest and amount of time for skin care is naive and can be frustrating for both patient and doctor.

A well-regarded dermatologist in my area provides patients with a formula or a recipe of skin care on preprinted forms. He tells his nurse to give Ms. Jones form number one, Mrs. Brown form number two and so on. Many of his patients have left him feeling they were being treated to cookie-cutter medical care.

Throughout this book I will share stories about my patients. This is to demonstrate how each individual presents unique and special problems not only from a purely medical point of view but from a personal one as well.

Helen

Helen, a successful architect in her forties, is beginning to show signs of aging from too much sun exposure. Having grown up in New Mexico with fair skin and a penchant for the outdoors, Helen has sun-damaged skin—fine lines, brown spots and dull skin. At first I thought Helen would benefit from the use of Retin-A. After getting to know her better, I decided against my initial plan. Why? Because Helen told me that she was either too tired or too busy to fuss with a product that required consistent nightly application for results. I therefore suggested a series of mild glycolic peels in the office.

The issue of compliance (following doctor's orders), played a role in how I designed Helen's cosmetic treatment program.

Helen enjoyed coming to the office for her half-hour treatment every other week. That was more her style. It was easier for her to make and keep an appointment than use Retin-A at home. For at-home care she used a moisturizer with SPF 15 during the day. With this routine her skin became softer and fresher. As a matter of fact, after about six months of treatments, she told me that a good friend had come up to her at a party and given her a compliment that almost anyone would like to hear: "You look too young!"

By getting to know her personal lifestyle and preferences, her likes and dislikes, Helen and I were able to devise a treatment plan that worked.

2. PATIENCE
Understand That Good Skin Comes from Careful Daily Attention

Lately it has become popular to allot a specific amount of time to achieve physical or emotional health: "better marriages in sixty days," "slimmer in three months," "smarter in one week." I have avoided this approach because I believe that beautiful skin can only be achieved through daily care and protection. Of course, I can tell you that a certain strength of glycolic acid can fade brown spots in eight weeks. I can explain how long it will take for Retin-A to reach its maximum effectiveness or how long a face-lift will last—but this is incomplete information.

You need to become a lifelong partner with your skin, and it will return the favor. You can keep your age a secret and look radiant—but not overnight—by following the right plan that works within the parameters of your lifestyle.

3. SELF-AWARENESS
Recognize That Wanting to Look Good Involves a Host of Psychological Issues

Much of this book is devoted to the pursuit of a better appearance. The difference between this book and many other "beauty guides" is that I am not simply offering advice to make you look better, I'm going further. I am committed to improving your well-being, your peace of mind, your comfort and self-confidence. Over the years I have learned that what people want to know about their skin translates into other important issues. It's just a matter of taking the time to remember that each patient is unique.

Norman

A man in his mid-forties entered my office about two years ago. He was conservatively dressed and appeared to be in good health except for mild obesity. His name was Norman, and he told me he had lived in a small town outside of Chicago. His work as a purchaser of gemstones and diamonds required trips to New York at least three times a week. As he told me about himself, I couldn't help feeling that Norman was sad and seemed burdened by something.

Norman had several moles on his body that he was concerned about and wanted me to examine. A full-body exam for moles is very thorough. Patients are completely undressed, and the doctor examines genitals, underarms and scalp. It requires delicacy and discretion on the part of the doctor.

A few of Norman's moles looked suspicious, so I scheduled an in-office surgery. Norman arrived a few weeks later and still seemed a bit distracted. During surgery, when a patient is awake, we sometimes speak to each other; some patients stay silent. Norman wanted to talk. He told me about his wife and two young children. Beside commuting, his work required him to travel extensively—Japan, South Africa, Spain.

"Do you enjoy traveling?" I asked.

Norman just sighed, and I dropped the subject.

Five days later Norman returned for a follow-up visit. His surgical sites were healing nicely. After he dressed, I asked him to step into my consultation room.

"Is there anything else I can do for you?"

"I'd like a blood test," Norman said.

"Anything in particular of concern?" I asked.

"Just a general one," Norman answered. It didn't seem that he wanted to talk.

When the blood test results came back, I noticed that Norman's liver enzymes were high and mentioned it to him.

"What could that mean?" he asked.

"Any number of things. It's hard to say. Do you drink?"

"Yes, I do," Norman said.

"How much?"

"Actually pretty heavily at times—when I travel, mainly." Norman cleared his throat, brushed a piece of thread off his pant leg, shifted in his seat and then looked at me. His face was full of anticipation.

"Did you do an HIV test?" he said finally.

"No. I would need your specific consent for that."

"I see.

"Would you like one?"

"Yes," Norman said. We made arrangements, and he hurried out.

I thought about Norman all week and was pleased when the test results came back negative.

Norman didn't react. He seemed miles away. Then he started talking.

"I wanted the test because . . . well, when I travel, I do drink quite a bit. And I have had several relations with women in these foreign countries. It's only when I'm drunk. Then I go home to my wife and feel awful. I love my family. I don't even know why I do this. I'm ruining my health. I'm risking everything I have."

Norman was the last patient that evening. He had never told anyone his secret. He said it was even difficult for him to admit it to himself. Somehow he felt I was the right person to tell. He said he trusted me.

Norman had been depressed for several years. He felt conflicted, guilty and alone. He said he wanted help.

I referred Norman to a psychiatrist whom I admired. A year of intensive therapy ensued, and Norman decided to stop drinking, to limit his travel to every other month and to discontinue his illicit relationships. The decisions were entirely his own.

About a year and a half after Norman's first visit, he returned to my office. He had lost weight and looked much more at ease.

After a few minutes of small talk Norman said, "I needed to talk to someone last year, and I am so fortunate that God sent me to you."

"You came to me for a mole check," I said, "but I was glad to help you any way I could."

"I had been hiding from myself for so long," Norman said. "I'm glad I trusted you."

When I think of Norman, I remind myself that people feel very vulnerable when they see a doctor. They take off their clothing, they answer personal questions, they are faced with complicated words and hard-to-understand concepts that affect their lives. This vulnerability should never be abused. It can be an opportunity, however, for a special kind of human interaction.

I encounter patients all the time who confide in me. I don't consider it a burden at all. It's part of the healing process. It's part of being a doctor. Literally and figuratively, a person's skin is just the start of who they are.

4. HOLISM
Beauty and Health Are Interconnected

Imagine yourself living in the age of the "cave man and woman." Your communication skills are limited, and just staying alive is a challenge—as you hunt and keep predators at bay. When it comes to finding a mate, what would you be looking for as the Stone Age single?

Scientists tell us that prehistoric people demonstrated a preference for symmetry over imbalance, a proportionate figure over obesity or a gaunt, undernourished look, and for signs of youthfulness—clear skin, a flexible physique. These outward manifestations indicated that our prospective partner was healthy, fertile, relatively clean and intelligent. Over thousands of years, things haven't changed much.

Perhaps this theory oversimplifies a complex issue, considering all the attributes that define modern beauty. That health and beauty are in some ways connected, however, is hard to dispute. My own definition of beauty begins with good health. Today, looking healthy doesn't necessarily mean looking twenty years old. I know many healthy-looking seventy-five-year-old men and women. In stark contrast, I have seen twenty-five-year-olds who look terrible, the result of a poor diet, bad habits and little interest in skin care.

Eating right for healthy-looking skin is critical. Foods rich in vitamins and fiber allow your body to restore and even correct the ravages of sun, dehydration and time. No amount of creams or plastic surgery can substitute for the critical daily intake of nutrients such as vitamins A, C and E, three of the most important building blocks of beauty.

Your standard for beauty should begin with good health. I will show you how to combine these two perfectly compatible ideals.

5. REALISTIC EXPECTATIONS
This Applies to Yourself and to Your Doctor

Comparing ourselves to others can inspire us to greater achievement, but it can lead to frustration, too, especially if we rely on media images as our role models. Why can't we be as thin as Kate Moss? Why can't our muscles bulge like Arnold Schwarzenegger's? We begin to believe that the illusion of perfection in movies and magazines is real. This leads to a cycle of anger and inadequacy. When a potential patient tells me that he or she is trying to "look like" someone else, a warning bell sounds in my head.

This comparison trap is especially dangerous when it comes to trying to look younger. A woman in her fifties can't expect to have the same face as a woman in her twenties. She can and should expect to look vibrant and healthy within an age-appropriate zone—perhaps five to ten years. Much depends on the starting point: a lot of sun damage or a little, a family history of early wrinkling or Hearty Skin.

In the following chapters I will provide you with important tips on choosing a doctor who is right for your needs. The number one principle regarding this search is finding a physician who you can trust. As a patient, your responsibility to have realistic expectations is equally important.

Achieving your personal best, regardless of your starting point, can bring enormous satisfaction. Appropriate, carefully planned treatments can restore a freshness and vitality to your skin. No one will mistake you for Cindy Crawford. You'll still look like you, only better.

6. MOTIVATION
Determine Why You Want to Look Better

You work long hours. You get up early in the morning so you can exercise. You sacrifice your leisure time in order to build stronger relationships with people who are important to you. Why? Each person's answer differs. The same is true when it comes to the desire to look more attractive.

In many cases, patients want to look younger or more attractive because they feel younger than they look. Others are embarking on new commitments or life challenges.

One New York plastic surgeon told me about a patient of his who wanted eyelid surgery although she was just thirty-four years old. The woman seemed to be an energetic, happy person with a loving husband and a fulfilling career. Why, wondered the plastic surgeon, was she interested in the surgical procedure?

The woman told him that she was planning to adopt a baby and didn't want to be mistaken for the child's grandmother. She was genuinely concerned about this issue. No one had suggested this idea to her. It came from the heart and out of a desire to begin her role as a mother in a positive way. She thought it would help her face the daunting task of motherhood and allow her to make the transition more easily. My colleague, a perceptive and discerning judge of character, told me that he believed her. In his judgment, the patient's decision was sound and well intended.

A few months after the surgery, with the adoption complete, the patient stopped in to see her doctor. She told him that she felt wonderful. She was confident and happy and loved being a mother. Both doctor and patient felt the decision was the right one.

Can a person want to look younger and more attractive for the wrong reason? This issue has sparked debate and controversy among feminist scholars as well as the medical community. In a recent dermatology journal, Dr. Eileen W. Ringel argued that providing cosmetic surgery for older people is "immoral." A doctor's first and only duty to a patient, Dr. Ringel believes, is to provide care that would lead to improved health, not a better appearance.

Opinions about body image, self-esteem and a person's reason for wanting to change his or her appearance abound, with no consensus in sight. Feminist authors such as Naomi Wolf have denounced society's imposition of beauty standards on women. Ms. Wolf claims that women have been manipulated by the media and controlled by others' ideas of perfection. Authors such as Nancy Friday and Camille Paglia claim that Ms. Wolf's point of view is victim-oriented and tends to patronize a woman's free will instead of celebrating her choices, sexuality and power. Yet another opinion comes from Harvard professor Nancy Etcoff, author of *Survival of the Prettiest*. Throughout history, human beings have been naturally attracted to others who are young and beautiful, according to Etcoff. Neither patriarchy, Madison Avenue nor any other societal construct originated the concept of physical attractiveness—soft, unblemished skin and a full head of hair for women, muscles and a strong jaw for men. An inherent biological appreciation for good looks has inspired the human species for centuries. Etcoff maintains, unlike Wolf, that there is really no one to "blame" for our desire to look attractive. It's just an inborn part of who we are.

My patients, rather than any academic discourse, have taught me the most about human nature and desires. An important issue facing a person looking for cosmetic improvement is knowing why you want to look better. Your awareness of your needs will make the experience more satisfying. You do not need to apologize for wanting to look better or younger. Only you know why you are trying to change. As Ms. Etcoff explains:

> *There is no such thing as a minor imperfection when it comes to the face or body. Every person knows the topography of her face . . . and body as intimately as a mapmaker. To the outside world we vary in small ways . . . In our mind's eye . . . a bad hair day, a blemish undermines our confidence.*

Some people search endlessly for perfection and never find it. The most flawless surgery leaves them feeling inadequate. One has to wonder whether an improved appearance is what they desire or whether something else is missing.

For the most part, however, people seeking plastic surgery understand that the procedure is neither magic nor an answer to all of life's problems. It is merely one of many avenues some of us pursue to live life more fully. Women and men have many reasons for wanting to look more attractive. Physicians must analyze the risk/benefit ratio without imposing their own values on someone else's decision about wanting to look better. Doctors can help a patient make informed decisions that will enhance the quality of her life and relationships, and assist in giving her confidence and peace of mind. Is that immoral? I think not.

Let me give you three examples that underscore the diversity of motivation.

Molly

Molly is a self-made millionaire, having invented and patented computer components which are used worldwide. Molly is confident, decisive and married to a man who is equally accomplished. Together they are a unique and dynamic pair. But Molly is a strong individual in her own right. She has been coming to my office regularly for nonsurgical treatments. After about two months of care, she stopped by and said while beaming with a devilish grin, "I have been accused of having a face-lift!"

We both laughed. Molly enjoyed fooling her friends. And it was clear that she was seeing me to please herself. She sets her own standards and lives by her own rules.

Mrs. Golden

A few years ago Mrs. Golden, who was well into her seventies, came to see me at my office with her adult son. When I asked about her medical history, she told me that she had been diagnosed with breast cancer and was told that it had spread to her lung. Sadly for her, the prognosis was not good. I asked if she was planning to have surgery, chemotherapy or radiation to treat her disease.

"No," she replied. "I've thought about it and decided to let nature take its course."

Her son could not persuade her. While it is every patient's prerogative to refuse treatment, I wanted her to understand fully the importance of her decision. She listened politely and smiled, but nothing I could say was going to change her mind. Then she told me that the reason she had come to my office was to have a tiny skin cancer called a basal cell carcinoma removed from her face. This lesion posed no threat to her health. It was in no way related to her breast cancer but evolved independently from sun exposure. The chance that it would spread anywhere else was remote. After I removed the tiny growth, she was scrupulous about keeping her appointments with me and caring for the scar so that it would heal without looking noticeable. She was most pleased with the results of her surgery and satisfied that she had taken care of the problem.

Mrs. Golden taught me a valuable lesson, one that many doctors overlook: One of the most precious gifts that a physician can give a patient is a sense of control over his or her body. Sometimes that's not possible because of the advanced stage of a disease, but sometimes even a little feeling of control can make a difference.

Mrs. Golden had bravely resigned to the fact that her breast cancer was advanced and not curable. She felt that she had lived a long and happy life, and she was not the kind of person who believed in miracles. Still, she wanted to do what she could to look better. Some people may think she was foolish. I think she was brave. She wanted to do something that in her eyes would improve the quality of the time she had left. I was honored to assist her.

Dr. Russo

Not long ago a thirty-four-year-old psychiatrist came to my office for a cosmetic consultation. "Dr. Russo" specializes in adolescent anxiety disorders. Like all doctors, she knows the necessity of a patient's absolute candor for proper diagnosis and care. I was therefore surprised at the events that unfolded during her first visit with me.

After some informal conversation, I took her medical history. "Any surgeries?" I asked.

"No," she answered.

I had previously noticed the telltale signs of a face-lift—small bilateral incisions along the front of her ears and a slight tightness in her face. I hadn't mentioned what I saw and expected the conversation to flow naturally.

"Any at all? Even a face-lift?" I asked again. She insisted, however, that she had not had any cosmetic surgery.

Her lack of honesty with me, and perhaps with herself, was troubling. It led me to believe that she will seek more and more procedures as time goes by. Did her reaction belie a certain ambivalence? Did she wonder, perhaps, whether she had done the right thing at the right time? Or was she afraid to admit that she simply wasn't satisfied? It seemed to me that Dr. Russo was a poor candidate for any type of cosmetic intervention.

All three patients, Molly, Mrs. Golden and Dr. Russo, came to me wanting to look better, but their reasons for wanting improvement varied. These stories illustrate that it is disingenuous to make blanket statements about the rightness or wrongness of anyone's wishes to improve his or her appearance. They also bring us back to the Six Virtues of Successful Skin Care that I have outlined.

Smart beauty is all about making the right choices at the right time. The passage of time changes our looks, but change can also be for the better—an opportunity to shine. The path to beauty is a process, not an endpoint. And like all journeys, the many routes, delayed departures and even some roadblocks make each trip different and interesting. Perhaps you have a medical problem such as diabetes or a heart condition that rules out extensive surgery such as a face-lift. I will show how you can improve what nature has provided by teaching you the fundamentals of skin care. You will learn about low-risk ways to smooth your skin and bring out your personal best. Maybe you just want to know how to buy the best moisturizer for your skin type. I will show you how to select the right products and, equally important, how to use them properly for maximum results. You will also learn how to correct mistakes such as overwashing and overusing creams and lotions that irritate your skin. I will teach you how to be an informed consumer of both over-the-counter goods and medical services.

The path to beauty will not just change the texture of your skin but will change you. Self-improvement is a highly personal endeavor. The rewards will mean the most to you, not someone else. You will develop an inner confidence that enhances the way you look and feel.

2

Aging Skin and How to Fight Back

Unlike internal organs, the skin ages right before our eyes. Changes are sometimes subtle, especially in people we see every day, including ourselves. When we meet an old friend after years of separation, however, we may notice a crinkled squint, a forehead line, a sprinkling of gray. To some these changes affirm the wonder of a long relationship. To others they symbolize how time touches all of us.

▇ More Than Wrapping Paper

As a dermatologist, I am particularly interested in the ways skin changes as we age and the importance of this phenomenon.

Is our skin just a sheet of wrapping paper holding our muscles and bones together? Not at all. It is the body's largest organ, a living, changing mantle of our self. What is happening within our body and our minds, good or bad, is often reflected on our skin. Simple phrases like "You're glowing" or "You're as white as a ghost" remind us that we can never completely hide our inner self. Goose bumps, hives, sweaty palms, a blush—all belie our insistence that we are calm and in control. Our skin speaks silently as it changes and reveals who we are.

Besides mirroring our feelings, the skin is itself a sensory organ which provides the pleasure of touch. During infancy, tactile expression between baby and caregiver affects physical and emotional development. The early experience of touch confers a special symbolic significance. Parent-child transactions also contribute to the development of self-esteem and body image. These interactions develop before a child can speak. The language is touch. Researchers have found that, like sleep and food, touching is vital to a baby's survival.

The skin also helps cool our body temperature by producing sweat. It insulates us from the cold as well. It creates vitamin D from sunlight. It protects us from injury and infection. It is literally the front line between the environment and ourselves.

■ Anatomy of Our Skin

Like an onion, the skin has many layers. The epidermis is the layer we actually see. Beneath that lies the dermis.

EPIDERMIS

The outermost layer of the epidermis is called the *stratum corneum*. It consists of a mosaic of cells called *keratinocytes*. These cells continually move upward from the bottom to the top layer of the epidermis while filling with keratin, an important skin protein. The journey upward from the lower layers of the epidermis to the upper layers takes about twenty-eight days. Biologically, cells of the stratum corneum are dead, but their function remains vital. The barrier they create forms the first line of defense against harm from water loss, invasion from toxic materials and damage from ultraviolet radiation (mainly sunlight).

Thickness, surface texture and level of hydration influence the appearance of our stratum corneum. Likewise, biological functions such as blood flow can make us look pale or flushed.

At the bottom layer of the epidermis you will find *melanocytes*. These cells are responsible for producing melanin, which imparts skin

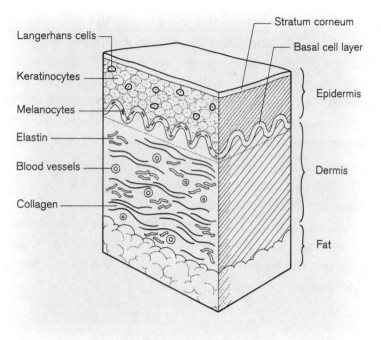

Langerhans cells

Keratinocytes

Melanocytes

Elastin

Blood vessels

Collagen

Stratum corneum

Basal cell layer

Epidermis

Dermis

Fat

ANATOMY OF THE SKIN

color. Your natural skin color as well as your tan are influenced by the activity of the melanocytes. Every person has the same number of
melanocytes regardless of race. The amount of melanin produced by the
melanocytes is what makes a person's skin darker or lighter. Melanocytes
produce and export melanin in packages called *melanosomes* that are
taken up by keratinocytes. Darker-skinned individuals have more active
melanocytes.

Langerhans cells in the epidermis play an important role in our immune system. They are actually the most distant outpost of surveillance
against invading micro-organisms, viruses and bacteria, even cancer. As
we age and our skin becomes damaged by ultraviolet radiation, fewer
Langerhans cells survive in the skin to provide immune protection.

DERMIS

Under the epidermis lies the *dermis,* which functions as a supporting frame for the outer portion of the skin. Structurally, small blood vessels, nerve branches and lymphatics are woven throughout this area.
Collagen is the most abundant protein within this layer. It is responsible

for the form, function and strength of our skin. Scientists describe the arrangement of collagen as bundles of interwoven strands. *Elastin fibers* are also contained within the dermis. This material allows the skin to rebound from deformities created by pressure or tension. *Ground substance* fills the space between collagen and elastin fibers. Its components play a vital role in the hydration of tissues since it carries with it a large volume of water.

Healthy collagen and elastin contribute to our skin's appearance, its relative firmness and plumpness. These characteristics translate into a youthful appearance.

ECCRINE GLANDS

These glands produce sweat and are found in almost all portions of the skin. Microscopically, these glands look like coiled tubes embedded in the dermis. Our body's complex temperature controls rely on eccrine glands to cool us off as the sweat they produce is evaporated from the surface of the skin. Eccrine glands are found in greatest abundance in palms, soles and *axillae* (underarms).

APOCRINE GLANDS

Associated with hair follicles in the dermis, these glands are found only in the underarm and ano-genital region and in a modified form in the ear canal, eyelids and breasts. Apocrine sweat, produced in small quantities, is broken down by skin bacteria and produces an unpleasant body odor.

SEBACEOUS GLANDS

These are present everywhere in skin except for palms and soles. They produce sebum, a waxy, fatty material. Sebaceous glands are most numerous on the face, forehead and scalp. Sebum secretion is controlled by hormones and reaches its maximum production at about twenty years of age and decreases about 28 percent per decade after that.

SUBCUTANEOUS FAT LAYER

Though not actually part of the skin structure, an important supporting component of skin is the *subcutaneous fat* layer. Fat serves to control temperature by reducing heat movement in and out of our body. The fat layer also cushions our internal organs and bones from trauma. From the standpoint of appearance, fat provides the body with its contours—be they attractive curves or unwelcome bulges.

Your Skin's Aging Process

TWO TYPES OF CHANGES

Two kinds of skin changes—*intrinsic* and *extrinsic*—illustrate how outside influences can add to or subtract from our appearance. Intrinsic aging refers to skin changes resulting from the chronological passage of time. Extrinsic aging is caused by exposure to the elements and results in prematurely aged skin. Intrinsic and extrinsic aging are two biologically independent processes.

Intrinsic aging occurs in everyone at a variable, genetically determined rate, often apparent between the ages of thirty and thirty-five. The changes brought about by intrinsic aging are relatively subtle and slow. There is a reduction in the density of hair follicles and oil glands, and also a loss of blood vessels, fat and collagen in the skin. The skin on the surface often remains smooth and unblemished despite these changes. For the most part the degenerative changes of intrinsic aging are irreversible.

Extrinsic aging results from exposure to the environment. It is a critical variable as to whether a person looks younger or older than another person of the same age. Long-term exposure to ultraviolet radiation—in particular sun exposure—is responsible for the majority of extrinsic skin problems. Damage to the skin caused by the sun is called photoaging. Too much time in the sun results in a leathery appearance, dilated blood vessels and spider veins *(telangiectases),* and mottled or spotty skin. Extremely sun-damaged skin can also become quite fragile, and even mild trauma can cause bruising.

Extrinsic damage from sun exposure accounts for most of our aged appearance. More than 90 percent of age-related changes to the face, back of the neck and "V" of the neckline, arms and back of the hands is caused by sun exposure. When does this damage take place? By some estimates, 75 percent of a person's lifetime ultraviolet exposure occurs by the age of eighteen, but the changes themselves are not obvious until middle age. Skin cancer, including melanoma, arises from sun damage as well.

The simplest way to see the difference between intrinsic and extrinsic aging is to look at sun-exposed areas of your body (hands, face, neck, forearms, for example) and compare those to non–sun-exposed areas (breasts, buttocks, inner arms). All these areas are chronologically the same age, but the differences in their appearance can be attributed to environmental factors.

The changes that take place within the skin on a microscopic level influence the way our skin looks to the naked eye.

With intrinsically aged skin, the epidermis thins. Elastin fibers may become coarser with age, and some may appear abnormal or eventually disappear. There is a reduced amount of collagen, but overall the skin remains smooth and unblemished.

By contrast, extrinsically aged skin is in much worse shape than intrinsically aged skin when viewed under the microscope. In some areas of the skin, the thickening of the epidermis makes the skin look rough and coarse. In other areas, the skin is thin and fragile. Langerhans cells are reduced in number and may contribute to the development of sun induced cancers. More degraded elastin is present as compared with intrinsically aged skin. There is also a greater loss of collagen.

Characteristics of Intrinsic Aging of Skin

Thin epidermis, imparting a transparent quality
Fewer hair follicles, sweat ducts and sebaceous glands
Decreased dermal collagen
Fine wrinkles
Paler color
Basically not reversible

Characteristics of Extrinsic Aging of Skin

Irregular pigmentation such as brown spots or uneven skin tone

Roughness/dryness

"Starburst" blood vessels, dilated capillaries

Deep wrinkles and furrows

Skin cancer

Breakdown of elastin

More significant decrease in collagen

Partially reversible with use of sunscreen, tretinoin (Retin-A), alpha hydroxy acids and antioxidants

YOUR SKIN AND THE SUN

What actually happens to our skin when it is exposed to the sun's damaging rays? The answers to this question may provide us with more clues to improve or even reverse aging skin.

Ultraviolet radiation injures the skin in many ways. Damage can occur after a single day at the beach or over a lifetime.

Ultraviolet radiation is divided into three wave bands: UVA, UVB and UVC. Only UVA and UVB reach the earth's surface. UVB causes an acute or immediate reaction in the form of redness and sunburn. When a person gets a sunburn, a chain of events within the skin takes place. UVB radiation results in the production of free radicals—molecular fragments that can damage healthy cells. One of the results of this exposure is the decline in the skin's capacity to repair itself.

Based on animal studies researchers believe that ultraviolet radiation also damages the skin's immune function. A single exposure to ultraviolet radiation can decrease the density of Langerhans cells for several days. Since those cells are a key component of a healthy immune system, immunosuppression may result from their injury.

Exposure to ultraviolet radiation not only compromises the immune function of the skin to which it is exposed but also throughout the body at sites distant from the exposed area. It also appears that increased amounts of melanin present in persons with darker skin do not completely protect the body from the sun's immunosuppressive effect. Likewise, sunscreen may not protect persons from the immunosuppressive effects of UV radiation. Therefore, sun avoidance should become an important goal even for persons with darker skin.

In contrast to UVB, the effects of UVA are not immediately apparent, but show up years later in the form of wrinkles and a loss of elasticity in the skin. Although UVB is still considered to be the major cause of skin cancer, it is no longer thought to be the only culprit. It also seems that UVA is involved in tumor formation, perhaps, in some cases, even as the primary agent.

Phases of Aging Skin

Consider the descriptions of the skin's appearance in the chart below and correlate them with your age. How does your skin measure up?

TYPE 1: NO WRINKLES, 20S TO 30S

EARLY PHOTOAGING
Mild changes in the color of the skin (age spots, liver spots)
No scaly bumps from sun exposure
Minimal wrinkles
Freckling is an early sign of skin damage in young persons

TYPE 2: WRINKLES IN MOTION, LATE 30S TO LATE 40S

EARLY TO MODERATE PHOTOAGING
Early freckles visible
Crow's feet begin to show
Small scaly bumps begin to grow
Parallel smile lines begin to appear on the sides of the mouth

TYPE 3: WRINKLES AT REST, EARLY 50S TO EARLY 60S

ADVANCED PHOTOAGING
Obvious blotches, spots, dilated capillaries and starburst blood vessels
Visible age spots and scaly bumps
Wrinkles visible even when not smiling or moving

(continued on next page)

(continued from previous page)

TYPE 4: ONLY WRINKLES, LATE 60S AND BEYOND

SEVERE PHOTOAGING
Yellow-gray skin
Skin cancers
Wrinkled throughout, no normal skin

■ ■

■ Fighting Back

After giving you all this unpleasant information about what happens to your skin as time goes by, I am now delighted to give you the good news. There are many things you can do to stave off these unwanted changes, especially with respect to photoaging. Avoiding excessive sun exposure should become the cornerstone of your skin care practice. Stay out of the sun when it is at its peak between 11 A.M. and 4 P.M. Use sunscreen with SPF 15 on your face every day. When you are planning to be outdoors, apply full-spectrum sunscreen of at least SPF 15 to any exposed areas of your body. Wear sun-protective clothing such as a long-sleeve shirt and pants, a broad-brimmed hat and sunglasses.

In addition to protecting your skin from the harmful effects of ultraviolet radiation, sunscreens may play a part in permitting the repair of photodamaged skin. In human studies, researchers found that the daily use of a sunscreen of SPF 17 reduced the number of new precancerous growths. Even more exciting was the fact that the likelihood of remission of precancerous growths was greater in the group that used sunscreen.

Probably the most potent remedy for both extrinsically and intrinsically aged skin is tretinoin. Most of the long-term studies have been done with Retin-A. After using Retin-A, skin biopsies from patients showed reversal of sun damage. Regular application over a ten- to twelve-month period resulted in an 80 percent increase in collagen formation. Daily use over four to six months improved fine and coarse wrinkling, skin texture and uneven pigment. Skin that is not sun damaged but shows signs of intrinsic aging can also benefit from Retin-A. Tests show that this type of skin becomes pinker and less wrinkled with regular use.

At the highest concentration, the maximum benefit is achieved in one year and can be maintained by less frequent applications. Unwanted side effects of these products include irritation and redness. Reducing the frequency and amount of application is the best way to resolve this problem.

Alpha hydroxy acids, which I will discuss in greater detail in upcoming chapters, can have a positive effect on photoaged skin. While no one is quite sure how or why alpha hydroxy acid works, researchers have noted that the epidermis and the dermis thicken and collagen and elastic fibers increase with the regular use of the appropriate strength and formulation of alpha hydroxy acid.

Antioxidants, especially those applied directly to the skin, also show promise in alleviating the signs of aging. Vitamins A, C and E appear to be those that are the most beneficial. In later chapters, I will describe how to use antioxidants for the best results.

While we all must face the fact that we are growing a bit older every day, it's good to know that scientific research and daily skin care can make a big difference in our appearance.

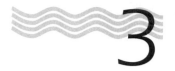

3

At-Home Care for
Skin, Hair and Nails

◼ Skin

You do it every day—washing, shaving, shampooing, clipping your nails, washing and drying your hair. Personal grooming, for most people, is a series of well-entrenched habits. Have you ever considered whether you are making the most of these daily rituals? Would you be willing to change your routine if doing so made your skin, hair and nails look more attractive and created a better-looking you?

When I see patients, I ask them about their routines. More often than you'd think, they're doing something wrong.

WASHING

Most adults over thirty commit one big mistake when it comes to washing: They do too much of it. A shower in the morning, another after the gym, maybe even one before bedtime. The average woman spends twelve minutes in the shower. That's too long. Cut your time in the shower to five minutes for your skin's sake.

Americans are personal hygiene maniacs—terrified of missing a daily bath, revolted by the thought of anything but a well-scrubbed, antiseptic body. Too much washing results not just in cleanliness but in itchy, irritated skin, particularly in the winter months.

I use the phrase "overwashed skin" to describe a large subset of people with dry skin whose problem comes from spending too much time in the tub or shower. Even people with oily skin can overwash. I'd estimate that over 75 percent of people who see me about dry skin don't know that overwashing is to blame for their itchy, irritated condition.

Lorraine

Lorraine, forty, is the senior vice president of a major brokerage house. She came to my office asking me to examine the white flakes and scales on her legs and arms. It took only a moment to make the diagnosis—dry skin. Lorraine looked perplexed. I'd even say she seemed disappointed.

"But, Doctor," she said, "I know this is a disease of some kind. Look at it again."

I obliged, if only to satisfy her.

"Lorraine, it's dry skin. If you want a technical name, it's called xerosis."

"But why? Why do I have xerosis? Is there something wrong with me?"

"You are using soaps that are too strong and washing too much," I responded.

We spent the next five minutes discussing the condition. I got the feeling Lorraine wanted me to tell her that she was allergic to something or had a disease that required a specific prescription ointment or pill. I advised her to change her skin care regimen, using milder cleansers and cooler water. She agreed to change her habits, but I still detected a dubious tone.

After about a month, Lorraine returned to my office for a follow-up appointment. Her skin was much smoother, and she had no flakes.

"I'm cured," she told me triumphantly. "What a strange disease!"

Overwashed skin not only looks terrible, but it can feel uncomfortable.

Mrs. Reeves

Mrs. Reeves arrived at my office impeccably attired in a fashionable mint-colored suit. Her hair was styled perfectly. She told me she owned an exclusive boutique on Madison Avenue. After a brief "hello," Mrs. Reeves sheepishly told me that she had been suffering from an itchy anus for four years.

While this might seem amusing to some people, this condition can be terribly annoying and anxiety provoking. I see many patients with this complaint—business tycoons, photographers, writers, lawyers, teachers. I actually overheard two businessmen discussing the issue across the aisle from each other on the Metroliner between New York and Philadelphia. The condition is so common it has a fancy Latin name—pruritis ani.

Ninety-five percent of the time, pruritis ani can be resolved without any medical intervention whatsoever. The only thing you need to do is avoid using soap in the affected area and reduce the amount of scrubbing. Mucous membranes are particularly sensitive to overwashing.

I reviewed Mrs. Reeves's daily hygiene routine. Like most people, she showered with hot water at least once a day, often twice a day. I was not surprised to hear that she was scrupulous about cleaning her anal-genital region with deodorant soap.

Many people can benefit from the following bathing tips:

- Avoid using a washcloth on delicate areas, especially the mucous membranes.
- Use medium-warm water in the shower. The cooler the better, but not too cold.
- For people with normal to dry skin, use DOVE UNSCENTED or BASIS FOR SENSITIVE SKIN on your body and either a soap-free cleanser or nothing at all on mucous membranes.

- If you tend to have oily skin, use a deodorant soap such as DIAL, SAFEGUARD or LEVER 2000 on any part of your body that tends to be oily—usually the back or chest. Do not use deodorant soap on your face. Legs and arms are hardly ever oily, even on people who tend to have oily faces, chests and backs. Use little or no soap on your arms and legs.

- Skip a shower. I am asking you to do—or rather not do—something that in our civilized society may seem appalling: Skip a shower for a whole day once or twice a week, especially in the winter. Instead of taking a shower or bath, gently wash your underarms, genital region and feet with a warm soft washcloth. Your skin's natural oil is one of the best protective barriers against dry skin. Allow your skin to produce and maintain that oil. Taking fewer and shorter baths and showers is the best way to prevent dry skin. Being careful about not washing too much is of particular importance to anyone over sixty. People in this age group need to bathe no more than three times a week, with light washing in between.

SOAP

Washing your face used to require two simple ingredients: soap and water. Today, the types of products available to complete this process have expanded to include cleansing bars, cleansing creams, astringents, toners, exfoliants and masks.

Soap contains "surfactants" that allow oil and water to mix. The oil and dirt, loosened from the skin, can be easily rinsed away. The more surfactant, the better the soap is at removing oil. Too much surfactant, however, can be quite harsh on many types of skin.

Most bars of "soap" today aren't soap at all. Take a look at the label on the next box of "soap" you buy. In many cases you won't even see the word "soap." Instead, manufacturers will call the product a "body bar," "beauty bar," "bath bar," a "deodorant bar" or a "moisturizing cleanser." If the bar you use for bathing does not claim to be a soap, it's probably a synthetic detergent. Even though the word detergent might make you think of harsh laundry powder, in the world of skin care, a synthetic detergent is often milder than soap. The technical name for a nonsoap cleansing bar is a "syndet bar." Products such as DOVE, OIL OF OLAY BEAUTY BAR and WHITEWATER ZEST are known as "Combars" because they are a combination of soap and a synthetic cleanser.

A lot of important information about soap is not available to the average consumer. For example, manufacturers do not list the pH of soaps on packaging. This is unfortunate since pH tells a lot about mildness or harshness. A soap's pH is a measurement of alkalinity or acidity on a scale of 0 to 14, with 0 being most acidic and 14 being most alkaline. For example, the pH of vinegar is 3.1. The pH of lye is 13. Healthy skin is naturally acidic, with a pH between 5.6 and 5.8. True soaps have a pH between 9 and 10. For people with even mildly dry skin, the pH of most soaps is too high. And it's not just dryness that results: Soap changes the composition of good bacterial flora and the activity of enzymes in the upper epidermis. Syndet bars have a pH adjusted to between 5 and 7, a good range for sensitive skin because it is so close to the skin's natural pH.

SOAP-FREE CLEANSERS

I am a big fan of soap-free cleansers, and my patients with sensitive or dry skin all praise them. They are gentle to the skin and effective for removing makeup and dirt. Many of us tend to focus on soap and cleansers without much thought about the other component of washing—water. The mineral content of water can vary from region to region around the country. In many areas of the country, minerals such as calcium, manganese and magnesium cause water to become "hard." Hard water can make washing and shaving unpleasant because it doesn't lather well and makes soap difficult to rinse. There have been reports of increased skin irritation and dryness with the use of hard water and soap as compared with soft water and soap. One interesting historical tidbit: during World War II, sailors on ships without the luxury of using freshwater for bathing used seawater but noticed that the soap did not foam. Soap-free cleansers were developed because of these problems. Besides mildness, another important benefit of using a synthetic detergent product instead of soap is that the type of water you use won't affect the way it works.

If your skin is oily and you think that you can change oil production

by washing it with a strong soap, think again. Your skin will not stop producing oil just because you washed oil away from the surface. Moreover,
many true soaps contain lards or fats that can block pores. What about
people with acne? In an experiment, a group of adolescents and young
adults with acne used a gentle "syndet bar" and another group used conventional soap. For the group using soap, the number of pimples increased. For the group using a syndet bar, the pimples decreased. The
conclusion to be drawn from this study is that cleansing the face with a
harsh soap won't make pimples go away and may even make things
worse.

RATING SOAPS

In another study rating the harshness of eighteen brands of soap,
DOVE, AVEENOBAR and PURPOSE were listed as the least irritating. ZEST,
CAMAY and LAVA were the harshest. I also recommend BASIS SENSITIVE
SKIN BAR SOAP, CARESS, TONE and OILATUM MOISTURIZING BAR.

If your skin is on the oily side or acne prone, try NEUTROGENA
CLEANSING BAR OILY SKIN FORMULA.

Regardless of what kind of skin you have and what kind of soap you
use, you will become uncomfortable at some point if you overwash. If
your skin feels itchy or dry, or looks red and irritated, before worrying
about an exotic disease, think about your shower/bathing habits because
they are most often to blame.

To wash your face with a soap-free cleanser, first dampen your face
with tepid water. Place a quarter-sized amount of cleanser in your palm
and then apply an even coat to your face. Massage gently with your fingertips. Rinse with tepid water, pat dry and moisturize.

Remember that mild cleansers don't make lather. They will not
leave you with that "squeaky clean" feeling, but that doesn't mean they
aren't doing a good job.

Types of Soap

TYPE	WHAT IT IS	COMMENTS
Acne	Sulfur, resorcinol, benzoyl peroxide or salicylic acid	For persons with Hormonally Reactive or Stress-Reactive Skin. Used correctly, can reduce breakouts. Use once in the morning: Splash face with tepid water, create a foam on your fingertips, then massage the skin lightly. Rinse thoroughly with tepid water. If skin becomes irritated, discontinue or use every other day. Abrasive acne scrubs should be avoided because they can cause irritation.
Castile	Olive oil used as main fat	Not superior to or more gentle than most other mild soaps. Can be drying if used too frequently, especially since many castile soaps contain other irritating ingredients.
Deodorant	Antibacterial agents	Many types contain an ingredient called tricolsan that eradicates various strains of bacteria. These have an alkaline pH that can cause skin irritation. It is not necessary to use a deodorant or antibacterial soap as your regular soap. It is useful, however, in preventing body odor; since body odor begins in the underarm, groin and feet, use deodorant soap in those areas only and a milder soap on other body parts. Oil-free deodorant soaps can be used as cleansers for body acne.
Facial and bath	No special ingredients; based on size of the bar	Do not be fooled into believing that a facial bar is gentler than a body bar.
French milled	Additives to reduce alkalinity	Reducing alkalinity theoretically will reduce irritancy, but check to see what other potentially irritating ingredients are in the product.
"Natural"	Aloe vera, vitamin E or herbs added	The number-one ingredient is either tallow, sodium laureate or another soap component. It is unlikely that the amount of added ingredients can be of any benefit and definitely will not make the soap milder. That is based on the pH.
Oatmeal	Ground oatmeal added	AVEENO is recommended. Avoid products with grainy texture.
Superfatted	Increased oil and fat; fat ratio up 10%	May contain ingredients such as lanolin and paraffin that moisturize. Works well for Overexposed Skin or very dry skin but should not be used more than once a day, preferably in the evening, followed by a moisturizer. Not necessarily milder.
Transparent	Glycerin and sucrose added	Usually milder than other soaps but are not preferred for the face. May clog pores of those who are acne-prone.

(Based on Zoe Draelos, *Cosmetics in Dermatology,* 2nd ed. New York: Churchill Livingstone, 1995.)

MILD SOAP-FREE CLEANSERS

For dry skin, try CETAPHIL CLEANSING LOTION, AVEENO CLEANSING LOTION or MOISTUREL SENSITIVE SKIN CLEANSER.

For oily skin, try CLINIQUE RINSE-OFF FOAMING CLEANSER, JOHNSON'S CLEAN AND CLEAR FOAMING FACIAL CLEANSER or NEUTROGENA OIL-FREE ACNE WASH.

COLD CREAM

Another category of cleansers include those that can be wiped off rather than rinsed off such as cold creams or cleansing creams. I recommend these products only for makeup removal. For most people they are too thick and greasy to be used as a cleanser.

To remove makeup, place the cold cream over the area of the face where makeup needs to be removed. If you are removing eye makeup, be careful to avoid getting the product into your eyes. Allow the product to "melt in" for a moment or two. By doing this you avoid having to rub your skin. Gently remove the cold cream and makeup in a circular motion. Rinse with warm water. If you were not able to remove all the makeup, try again. If you find cold cream too heavy and greasy, as many women do, try CLINIQUE CRYSTAL CLEAR CLEANSING OIL.

Use a cotton-based tissue to remove the makeup. New low-irritancy tissues are available through Purely Cotton Linters, Inc., on the Internet (www.purelycotton.com). Unlike cotton balls, they leave no residue on the skin.

ASTRINGENTS AND TONERS

I am not a big fan of astringents and toners. For persons with sensitive skin, these products have the potential to irritate and have only minimal cosmetic benefit. Most women over thirty-five do not need astringents or toners. The claims that these products will "tighten" your skin are misleading. According to one expert, astringents used to be of some value when harsh soaps and hard water made rinsing soap residue difficult. Since this is not the situation in most homes, astringents have little place in your already overstocked bathroom. If your skin feels as if it needs a little more cleansing after you have washed it, apply a mixture of one part lemon juice with ten parts water and rinse thoroughly with warm water.

Most people do not need to bother with exfoliants. Newer formulations of alpha hydroxy acid have replaced the need for exfoliation among people with Overexposed Skin. Persons with acne-prone skin should use mild alpha hydroxy or salicyclic acid products.

FACIAL MASKS

A twice-monthly treatment with a facial mask can help certain types of skin look a little better. While you can get a face mask at a salon, many over-the-counter products are just as good at half the price. I prefer facial masks over exfoliants, astringents or scrubs because they tend to be milder and involve less mechanical manipulation of the face such as scrubbing, scraping and rubbing.

For persons with dry or aging skin, wax, paraffin or other moisturizing ingredients are recommended. Professionals usually heat the mask ingredients slightly before application, because this enhances the moisturization process. Try the BODY SHOP INTENSE MOISTURE MASK.

For persons with acne-prone skin, masks with earth based materials such as mud or clay work best. Paula Begoun, author of *The Beauty Bible,* recommends the use of a MILK OF MAGNESIA mask for persons with oily skin. My patients report that it is a soothing treatment for skin that tends to break out. Try ALPHA HYDROX PURIFYING CLAY MASQUE.

BODY MOISTURIZING

After washing, moisturize while your skin is still damp, starting with your shoulders and working your way down to your feet. Remember that products that may seem sticky or thick in the jar won't stay that way once they mix with your damp skin. Applying moisturizer to damp skin will also prevent the water still on your skin from evaporating. This will leave you feeling more comfortable and allow for better absorption and a more even coating.

Simple, inexpensive products work fine.

Some Recommended Body Moisturizers

NIVEA SKIN THERAPY with vitamin E

AVEENO MOISTURIZING LOTION (a thinner consistency that is perfect for acne-prone skin)

EUCERIN LOTION (good for drier skin)

CETAPHIL MOISTURIZING LOTION (good for most skin types and especially good for people with eczema; perfect for the whole family)

OVERRATED AND NOT RECOMMENDED

LUBRIDERM

KERI LOTION

IF YOUR BUDGET ALLOWS

KIEHL'S ALOE MASSAGE CREAM is good for allover body softening and is especially soothing for pregnant women. Call 800-KIEHLS-1 or 2. For cracked skin try AQUAPHOR OINTMENT.

LOW-BUDGET ALTERNATIVES

Olive Oil and CRISCO. Of course, they don't smell great, but they also don't contain a lot of needless fragrance or additives, either. Because oils can be quite greasy, you may wish to gently wipe off any excess with a soft towel before dressing.

MICROPOWERED MOISTURE

A new group of products on the market called "micropowered moisturizers" deliver oil in a pump spray. They usually contain mineral oil and some fragrances. Their best features are that you don't need to get your hands greasy, they're easy to apply and because they are in a pump, you can get to hard-to-reach areas. ST. IVES BODY LOTION MIST and AVON'S SKIN SO SOFT MOISTURIZING SPRAY are two examples.

SCENTED CREAMS

Expensive body creams and moisturizers from department stores, especially designer-scented creams, have never impressed me. They tend to cost at least five times as much as drugstore products. Most have too much fragrance. Many are sticky and difficult to apply. Not only can they be irritating but some pose specific risks to sensitive individuals. For example, perfumes and body creams with oil of bergamot (SHALIMAR, for example) can cause a serious skin reaction in some people when they are exposed to sunlight. This is also true of certain citrus-based fragrances. Because the ingredients of a fragrance are generally not listed, you should probably avoid using new products if you tend to have sensitive skin.

Before purchasing any scented cream, apply a small amount to your inner arm and wait about forty-five minutes to see if you develop any irritation from it.

If you enjoy wearing a scent, purchase some essential oils from a health food store and try this: Mix a few drops of the oil into a handful of standard unscented body moisturizer and apply. Lavender is a very nice choice. Cinnamon and rose are not recommended for sensitive people. If you don't have a reaction, you will know you can tolerate that particular scent.

ALPHA HYDROXY ACID PRODUCTS

Alpha hydroxy acid products help very dry skin and need to be used on a regular basis for the best results. LAC HYDRIN, available by prescription, is a 12 percent concentration of neutralized lactic acid and helps in cases of severely dry skin. LAC HYDRIN FIVE, available over the counter, has a 5 percent concentration.

African-American skin can sometimes become ashy. The skin dries, flakes and sometimes thickens. Ashiness can impart a grayish tone to the skin. LAC HYDRIN offers effective relief for this problem.

SPECIAL TREATMENTS FOR DRY DARK PATCHES

I see a lot of people who are concerned about dark skin on their elbows and knees and ankles. These parts of your body can often become very dry. Excessive keratin can build up on these parts of your body and create dark patches.

To alleviate this problem, take a five- to ten-minute bath in warm water. Add two tablespoons of mineral oil to the bath. After soaking in the tub, gently rub the elbows and knees with a damp washcloth. If the areas are especially rough and dry, use M.D. FORMULATIONS BODY SCRUB.

After your bath, apply cut lemon to the elbows, knees and ankles, then rinse with cool water. Follow up with an emollient moisturizer such as VASELINE, AQUAPHOR OINTMENT or EUCERIN CREAM. Use LAC HYDRIN daily to keep the patches in check.

DRYING YOUR SKIN

Use a clean soft towel that has been washed in fragrance-free, dye-free detergent and dried without any fabric softener or "static-free" cloths. Fragrances and dyes in detergents can irritate sensitive skin. (See chapter 7, Environmentally Sensitive Skin, for more information.)

Make sure that you thoroughly dry between your toes and in the groin area to reduce the risk of a fungal infection. All other body parts should be patted gently and air dried.

Hair

While there are many seemingly important functions of hair among mammals (warmth, cushioning, sensory perception, camouflage), the overriding function among humans is sexual attraction. Perhaps that explains our concern with and attention to the cluster of "tough fibrous proteins" that we call hair.

Hair can be a trademark or send a signal about our personality. Albert Einstein's shock of unruly hair leaves us with the indelible impression of a brilliant and slightly absentminded scientist. Cleopatra's image would not be complete without the thick ridge of bangs framing her kohl-lined eyes.

The adage "The grass is always greener on the other side of the fence" applies perfectly to the way we tend to view our hair. Those with curls will do almost anything for straight hair. And those with straight hair endure hot rollers, curling irons and permanents for curls. We long for more of it on certain parts of our body and do everything we can to banish it on others. We curse the first gray hairs as an insistent herald of old age. We layer and trim. We tease. We never tire of looking for ways to enhance our hair.

Out of this preoccupation a billion-dollar hair care industry has been spawned. Silky, shiny, lustrous, thick, manageable, healthy hair are the promises that hair care companies make. Are they telling the truth? And what can you do to keep your hair looking good?

Regardless of your hair color, thickness and length, it is subject to damage from excessive or improper drying, combing, styling, dyeing and perming. Another enemy is the environment—sunlight, wind, seawater, chlorinated pool water and air pollution.

HAIR ANATOMY

Your hair is made up of the cuticle, cortex and medulla. The cuticle is the hair's outermost layer. Beneath the cuticle is the cortex, which provides our hair color. The innermost hair structure is the medulla.

Like the epidermis, the cuticle is made up of overlapping cells assembled like fish scales. Well-maintained healthy hair has smooth, even cuticles. Too much perming, processing or trauma can cause this orderly row of cells to break down, resulting in weak, dull hair.

Hair itself is made of a fibrous protein called keratin. The average human scalp has one hundred thousand strands of hair, with blond hair the most numerous followed by brunettes and then redheads.

Hair grows in a cyclical phase. There is a period of active growth, followed by a resting period. During the active period, your hair grows about one-third to one-half inch per month. At any one time 85 percent of your hair is in this growth phase. Some of the hairs on your head are resting, some are growing and others are somewhere in the middle.

One of the most remarkable properties of hair is its hardness, which is similar to stainless steel's. Hair fibers pressed between the jaws of a stainless steel vise leave a slight indentation. Despite its strength, hair is delicate. It should be handled gently since it is virtually impossible to repair hair once it has been damaged. The best you can hope for is a temporary fix with conditioners and other treatments. While these products

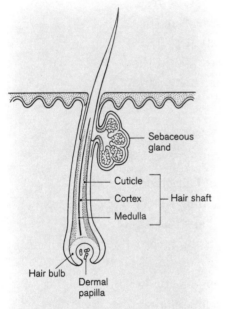

ANATOMY OF THE HAIR FOLLICLE

can do wonders for the appearance of your hair, they can't change its essential condition. For that you need to wait until new hair grows in.

SUN PROTECTION

Protecting your hair from the sun is also wise. Excessive exposure to ultraviolet radiation causes brittleness and loss of shine and can affect color. Some hair products claim to provide sun protection, but to date there is no standardized method of measuring this. Any product that is rinsed out of the hair will do nothing to protect your hair from the sun. For the best cover, use a breathable but densely woven hat or scarf.

SHAMPOO

What makes your hair dirty? Oils from your sebaceous glands, debris from the scalp and dirt from the atmosphere. Active individuals usually find their hair becomes dirty after a strenuous workout because of sweat residue. Humid weather can make almost anyone's hair sticky and heavy.

It was not until the 1950s that hair shampoo was widely used. Before that, people used plain soap. The biggest selling point for shampoo was its ability to rinse efficiently without residue.

One of the most common shampoo ingredients is lauryl sulfate. This ingredient is good for coarse or oily hair. It cleans well but provides little conditioning. By contrast, laureth sulfate provides better conditioning and also cleans well, so it is recommended for normal to dry hair. Read the labels carefully when considering your purchase.

The shampoo industry goes to great pains to develop shampoo that produces an abundance of suds and foam. It does this not because suds improve the product but because marketing executives know that creamy sudsiness creates a "signal" to which consumers respond *(buy!)*. In other words, more suds, more sales.

I have two problems with this issue: More suds don't make a shampoo work better and may even be very drying to certain types of hair, and the chemicals used to create the suds can be hazardous to your health. *Diethanolamine (DEA)* boosts lathering, but has been associated with liver cancer. The Federal Drug Administration has alerted consumers that DEA-related compounds (oleamide DEA, lauramide DEA and cocamide DEA) show an association with cancer in laboratory animals. *Crotein Q (steryl trimonium hydrolyzed collagen),* which is added to shampoos to increase performance, can cause hives, especially among sensitive persons.

OPTIMAL SHAMPOOING

1 Brush or comb your hair before getting into the shower.

2 Wet hair thoroughly with warm water.

3 Pour about two quarter-size amounts of shampoo into your hand.

4 Apply the majority of the shampoo to the roots of your hair, especially at the front of the scalp and at the back of the neck.

5 Lather in with a gentle circular motion, being careful not to scratch your scalp with your nails.

6 Instead of a second application, spend the time working the shampoo in. Unless your hair is very oily, you do not need to repeat the shampoo process.

7 Rinse with cool water, making sure to remove all residue. Tip for oily hair: Apply the shampoo with a thick-toothed comb before you wet your hair. Wait three minutes and then wet your hair. A great oil buster.

Remember that your hair is weaker and subject to breakage when it is wet. Be careful when combing it.

Shampoo Recommendations

NORMAL HAIR (FOR DAILY USE)

PHYTOMIEL WITH HONEY CORNFLOWER EXTRACTS by Laboratories Phytosolba

L'ORÉAL HYDRAVIVE GENTLE SHAMPOO for NORMAL EXTRA BODY

SENESCIENCE ENERGY SHAMPOO

REVLON FLEX BALSAM AND PROTEIN MOISTURIZING SHAMPOO

OILY HAIR

It is difficult to find shampoos specifically recommended for oily hair. Look for other key words such as "deep cleansing" or "for fine, limp hair." Too much conditioning and too many protein-based ingredients can add to the oily problem and should be avoided. Try the following products for oily hair.

GOLDWELL'S KERASILK SHAMPOO

VIDAL SASSOON STYLIST CHOICE A EXTRA BODY FOR FINE OR THIN HAIR

PANTENE PRO-V PRO VITAMIN CLARIFYING SHAMPOO

CLAIROL HERBAL ESSENCE FOR OILY HAIR

DRY HAIR

If your hair is very dry, apply a tablespoon of plain yogurt after washing once a week. Leave it in for a minute and rinse.

AGREE HYDRATING FORMULA FOR DRY, DAMAGED, OR PROCESSED HAIR

VIDAL SASSOON ULTRA CARE MOISTURIZING ALL-IN-1 FOR DRY, PERMED, OR COLOR-TREATED HAIR

Shampoo-and-Conditioner-in-One Products

I disagree with beauty experts who do not recommend shampoo-and-conditioner-in-one products. If you select the correct product, you can save time and money and end up with soft, manageable hair, especially if you don't have time for more than wetting, sudsing and a quick rinse. Shampoo-and-conditioner-in-one products also work well for people whose hair gets "bogged down" with a separate conditioner.

NORMAL TO DRY HAIR

KISS MY FACE KISS AND GO SHAMPOO AND CONDITIONER IN ONE

NORMAL TO OILY HAIR

PANTENE PRO-V SHAMPOO PLUS CONDITIONER FOR FINE HAIR

SUAVE SHAMPOO PLUS CONDITIONER REGULAR FORMULA

PERT PLUS SHAMPOO. This shampoo can be a little harsh, so I wouldn't use it more than three times a week, but it does give hair a body boost.

Conditioners

Most hair can benefit from conditioning to improve manageability, increase shine and mend split ends temporarily. (There is no permanent way to repair split ends.) People with oily hair may need to condition less often. Once a week is usually enough. If your hair and scalp tend to be dry, once a week massage conditioner into your scalp at night and leave on. Wash and rinse in the morning.

Look for the following ingredients, depending on your hair problem.

CHEMICALLY PROCESSED HAIR (DYED OR PERMANENT WAVED)

Look for "Quaternary ammonium" compounds which increase shine and improve manageability.

INFUSIUM 23 LEAVE-IN TREATMENT ORIGINAL FORMULA FOR DAMAGED HAIR

VO FINE THICKENING CONDITIONER

SPLIT ENDS

Look for "Hydrolized proteins" which penetrate and temporarily strengthen the hair shaft. The source of the protein is not very important.

SUAVE CONDITIONER WITH BALSAM AND PROTEIN

TRESEMMÉ EUROPEAN BODY-BUILDING CONDITIONER

REVLON FLEX BALSAM AND PROTEIN EXTRA BODY CONDITIONER

If you don't mind the mess, you can apply beaten eggs, milk or gelatin to your hair and then rinse.

OILY HAIR

REDKEN PHINAL PHASE ULTRA LIGHT CONDITIONER

L'ORÉAL FORTAVIVE CLEAN RINSE CONDITIONER

Clarifying Shampoo

Once a week, wash your hair with a clarifying shampoo to remove the residue left behind by hair treatment products.

NEUTROGENA SHAMPOO

SUAVE DAILY CLARIFYING SHAMPOO

REGIS CLEARLY CLEAN SHAMPOO

To clarify oily hair: Massage one part apple cider vinegar and one part water into the scalp several times a week before you shampoo. Don't rinse. Your hair will look shiny.

COMMON HAIR PROBLEMS

Dandruff and dandruff shampoos. Dandruff is the overproduction of cells on the epidermis of the scalp that clump together. Shampoos with zinc pyrthione (ZPT) and pyroctone olamine fight dandruff. Experts have found that the latter ingredient works better. The old standard HEAD AND SHOULDERS is an effective dandruff fighter.

Tar-based shampoos treat dandruff as well, especially if your hair and scalp tend to be oily. IONIL T or NEUTROGENA T/GEL are popular and effective tar-based shampoos. If you have light hair, tar shampoos can discolor your hair and are not recommended. Instead, try a prescription brand shampoo called NIZORAL. I do not recommend the long-term use of tar-based shampoos. Overusing them may result in pimples on the scalp and neck. Use only once or twice a week for a two-month period. If you are not getting effective relief in that time period, see your dermatologist.

Besides using the right products, you need to use the right technique. After applying the tar-based or medicated shampoo, massage thoroughly to ensure it contacts the scalp—not just the hair—and wait at least five minutes before rinsing.

Like your skin, your scalp can become flaky, dry and itchy, especially during the winter months. Low humidity, wearing hats and too much hair washing all contribute to your scalp problem. To combat this problem, moisturize with a hot oil treatment such as ALBERTO VO5 HOT OIL TREATMENT. You can economize by using warmed olive, avocado or walnut oil. Apply with your fingers and gently massage the roots. Wrap your hair in a soft towel or shower cap for about fifteen minutes, then rinse with a gentle protein-based shampoo. Use warm, not hot water.

Another option for people with dandruff is the use of alpha hydroxy acid shampoos. Use an AHA shampoo once a week, and if you do not experience any irritation, increase to twice a week. These products will do two good things: strip away grime and retain moisture. Try MURAD'S

ADVANCED SCALP TREATMENT (800-915-0230) or ABBA'S ALPHA HYDROXY HAIR AND BODY CLEANSER.

Is it just dandruff? Flaking, redness and itching on the inner portion of your eyebrows or sides of the nose are signs of an inflammatory condition called sebhorreic dermatitis whose cause is unknown. It can be treated with NIZORAL SHAMPOO, tar-based shampoos and steroid creams.

Psoriasis and eczema can mimic dandruff as well because they create flakes on the skin. These conditions are more difficult to treat, and it is recommended that you see a dermatologist if your "dandruff" persists despite medicated shampoos.

HAIR DRYING

Do you remember the giant metal bonnets women sat under in the beauty parlor while their "set" dried? Since the 1970s, the blow-dryer, immortalized in *Saturday Night Fever*, has become a staple of household hair care equipment. Like any convenient gadget, however, it can be used incorrectly—with damaging results. To dry hair the right way:

1 After washing and combing your hair, dry it gently with a soft towel and comb again. Don't use the blow-dryer until your hair is at least halfway air-dried. You will save time and prevent your hair from drying out. This is true even for oilier hair.

2 Be careful not to lean the nozzle against your scalp.

3 Protect your hair with a stay-on conditioner or other styling aid. Try NEUTROGENA HEAT SAFE INSTANT HEAT ACTIVATED HAIR TREATMENT.

4 Switch to a cooler setting when your hair is almost dry.

OTHER HAIR CARE PRODUCTS

The hair care products industry faced major changes in the 1980s when consumers started clamoring about health hazards and performance claims. According to analysts in the field, the manufacturers "undertook the radical reformulation of products" during this era.

Hair spray. These products rank second to shampoo in the hair care market. The first generation of hair sprays were nothing more than aerosolized shellac. Today, shellac has been replaced with conditioners and other hair-friendly ingredients. In general, mid-price-range hair sprays are usually the best to use. That's because more expensive sprays often contain a lot of unneeded fragrance. Try the following:

FINESSE HYDRATING SILK PROTEIN ENRICHED HAIR SPRAY by Helene Curtis, which has fragrance, but it is last on the list of ingredients
AUSSIE MEGA STYLING SPRAY by Redmond
SPRITZ FORTE by Sebastian International

Gels. These popular hair cosmetic products are almost identical to hair spray except for their formulation and packaging. Alcohol-free gels are recommended to avoid drying out the hair. In general, hair gel poses little risk for irritancy.

SOME RECOMMENDED STYLING PRODUCTS:
AVEDA BRILLIANT FORMING GEL is good for more dramatic styling. Not too heavy. Provides finish and shine.
ALBERTO VO5 CONDITIONING HAIRDRESSING is a classic. Contains no alcohol, and it conditions while you style.
SEBASTIAN STYLING MUD, which, as the name implies, is not exactly a gel, but it is good for styling, grooming and smoothing flyaway hair.
KIEHL'S SHINE 'N LITE GROOM is great for dry or normal hair. Works on frizzy or straight hair to manage and give body.

Kitchen hair. Mayonnaise provides great conditioning and moisture, especially because it is so rich in eggs. Beer comes in handy as a setting lotion, and it actually doesn't smell so bad after a minute or two. If your hair is very dry, cooking oils coat beautifully. You can use a mixture of water and gelatin as a setting gel.

Application Tip

The biggest mistake women make when applying styling products is starting from the roots and working down the hair shaft. Bend over and flip your hair. Put the hair product in the palm of your hand and blend in with your other hand. Start at the ends of the hair and work your way up to the scalp.

Mousse. Try mousse if gels are too heavy for your taste but you still want a little boost. Mousse is used in the same way as gel but is generally less sticky and spiky. Be sure not to put too much mousse on your hair as it will weigh it down. A dollop about the size of a half-dollar should do it for most people. VIDAL SASSOON MOUSSE is recommended.

COLORING YOUR HAIR: IT'S HUE!

One out of four women regularly use hair dye. While some women just like to change their color for fun, most use dye to cover the dreaded gray. Silver or gray hair can crop up at almost any age. You cannot turn gray overnight, but you can develop gray hairs from certain illnesses, including stress-related episodes. When hair turns gray from aging, it will never return to its original color. When hair turns gray from diseases, such as endocrine disorders, malaria and influenza, it has a chance of returning to its original color once new hair can grow in.

Fundamentally, hair turns gray because pigment cells become inactive. This internal process cannot be slowed down or terminated. Genetics plays a major role in gray hair.

Types of hair dyes. Used correctly, hair dye can not only improve the color of your hair but add the appearance of depth and fullness. The basic principle behind all hair dye is the penetration of the cortex of the hair itself. The more deeply the dye is penetrated, the more lasting the dye will be. There are five different types of hair coloring.

    ● Temporary coloring with textile dyes. As the name implies, temporary coloring doesn't last. With one or two shampoos, it's gone. You can't lighten your hair with a temporary color, but you can brighten or enrich your existing color. Temporary coloring, also called a "color rinse," does not penetrate through the cuticle of the hair unless the hair is very damaged from chemical treatments. It is great for people who can't make up their minds!

● Gradual coloring with metallic salts. The most common brand of gradual coloring is GRECIAN FORMULA, which promises to eradicate gray hairs over a period of time so that no one will notice. Avoid gradual coloring. It doesn't provide good color, it damages hair and it will interfere with permanent waves and permanent hair dye.

● Semipermanent coloring. Semipermanent dyes cover gray, add highlights and tone down color in a manner that is more subtle than more permanent products. They add tone rather than drastic color changes. The dye is generally washed out in four to six shampoos. Recommended for people who have less than 30 percent gray. Semipermanent coloring is less likely than permanent dyes to cause an allergic reaction and therefore is the choice for people with Environmentally Sensitive Skin.

● Permanent coloring. The most popular form of hair coloring in the United States is permanent hair dye. An alkaline solution swells the hair's cuticle, allowing the dye to penetrate into the cortex. Coloring the hair causes only mild damage to the cuticle, but too frequent or careless applications can lead to breakage. The advantages of permanent hair dyeing are that it lasts and that it comes in a variety of shades which allow you to cover gray or lighten hair.

Paraphenylenediamine dyes (PPDAs) in these colorings may cause allergic contact dermatitis. Some people who are allergic to PPDAs are also allergic to ingredients in semipermanent dyes.

● Natural coloring with henna. Some women prefer henna dyes because of the belief that they are "natural" substances. Actually, most henna dyes are synthetic henna-type products. Henna stains rather than dyes the hair and is used on the nails and skin in some countries. Henna comes from crushed leaves and contains a chemical called lawsone. Laboratory observations indicate that lawsone can cause anemia in some individuals.

Henna does not cover gray hair well, nor can it lighten hair. Henna can cause the hair to become brittle and stiff, so most modern formulations include chemicals to offset these problems. When chemicals are added, the product is usually called a compound henna. It is best used for a person with medium brown or light brown hair who wants a richer cast.

Keeping color vibrant. Keep your hair color fresh and your hair as healthy as possible by following these basic rules:

- Wash your hair as infrequently as possible.
- Use cool water and a cool setting on your blow-dryer.
- Use shampoo and conditioner formulated for dyed hair such as REDKEN COLOR EXTEND or IRRADIANCE SHAMPOO AND CONDITIONER.
- Avoid sun exposure as much as possible. When in the sun, wear a hat or scarf.
- Rinse or lightly wash your hair with cool water after swimming in a pool.
- Handle your hair gently, avoiding any tugging or pulling.
- Don't perm your hair and dye it at the same time. If you both perm and dye your hair, perm first, wait ten days and then dye it.
- When "touching up" dyed hair, concentrate on the newly grown "roots" and less on the already dyed hair to avoid further damage.
- If you bleach your hair, wash after bleaching and not before.
- Follow all package instructions, especially the warning to patch test a small portion of the hair to avoid an allergic reaction.

Hair Removal

WET SHAVING

Shaving is the most common form of hair removal, probably because it is the quickest and most convenient. Nicks, ingrown hairs, scrapes and incomplete hair removal are the most common problems associated with shaving. These shaving annoyances and others can be avoided by following these tips.

Men

1 Use plenty of warm water to moisten the skin and soften beard stubble. The ideal situation is to shave after your shower.

2 Next, apply a not-too-greasy facial moisturizer. I recommend NIVEA HEALTHY SKIN products. If your skin tends to be very oily, wash your face with a nondeodorant soap.

3 Apply a conditioning shave preparation. The most effective is AVEENO THERAPEUTIC SHAVE GEL, which is great for sensitive skin because it is fragrance-free. Other good products are CLINIQUE SHAVE ALOE GEL, AVEDA'S SHAVE EMOLLIENT and KIEHL'S "CLOSE SHAVERS" SHAVE CREAM. Let these products soak in for at least three minutes, preferably five minutes. Shaving creams work by hydrating the whiskers, making them easier to cut.

4 Shave in the direction of the whiskers. On your neck the direction of the whiskers may change abruptly—and several times—so look carefully. In general, you should shave down the cheeks and up the neck.

5 Try to shave slowly and carefully, going over each area once instead of repeatedly.

6 Change blades regularly because dull blades do not shave well. Do not let blades rest on any surface. Either recap or place with the blades facing up.

7 After shaving your face, remember to lubricate the skin with a moisturizer.

In a pinch, any type of hair conditioner can effectively soften stubble and keep the underlying skin from nicking.

For men with curly beard hair, ingrown hairs can result in a condition known as pseudofolliculitis barbae. Alpha hydroxy acid products can help prevent this condition because they exfoliate dead skin, which interferes with outward growth. MD FORMULATIONS BODY SCRUB is a good choice, and it works well on other rough spots such as the feet and elbows. AQUA GLYCOLIC ASTRINGENT helps straighten hair and can reduce ingrown hairs. If you have a tendency to develop ingrown hairs, use a single-bladed razor instead of one with double blades. And remember to rinse your razor frequently while shaving.

Women

The above tips apply to women with some additional advice:

● Be extra careful when shaving shins and knees because bony areas are more easily nicked.

● To avoid irritation, opt for more frequent, less close shaves.

● While it is important to soak your skin before shaving, don't soak for more than five minutes. After that, your skin can wrinkle from too much water and create an uneven surface for shaving.

Since legs tend to become drier than faces, it's important to give your legs special attention after shaving. Moisturizers with any fragrance or alcohol tend to sting or irritate newly shaved skin. I have found that VASELINE PETROLEUM JELLY CREAMY FORMULA WITH VITAMIN E is an excellent nonirritating "after-shave" moisturizer for legs, especially during the winter months. Well-prepared studies have shown that petroleum jelly actually aids in healing any cuts on the skin, an added bonus if you nicked your legs. While your legs are still wet, apply a quarter-sized amount to each. Allow it to absorb before dressing.

ELECTRIC SHAVING

Some people prefer shaving with an electric shaver. In general, you will not get as close a shave with dry shaving as you do with wet. This method is usually quicker than other methods but is generally less than optimal. Some people prefer electric shaving because it is less likely to cause abrasion. Electric shaving is not recommended for underarms or the bikini area because it can be irritating.

Tips for Electric Shaving

● Clean the face first with warm water and a gentle facial soap.
● Make sure the skin is dry.
● Moisturize afterward.

PLUCKING

Three items are essential for successful plucking: good tweezers, adequate light and a mirror for areas such as the eyebrows.

Plucked hair stays away longer than shaved hair. Plucking is best reserved for small areas. The biggest risk with plucking is ingrown hairs and the failure of hair, especially the eyebrows, to regrow. I have seen many female patients who complain about sparse eyebrows as the result of overzealous plucking years before. Remember that your eyebrows will become less dense as you grow older, so you should be very conservative about how much hair you remove.

For optimal plucking results:

Wash the tweezer with liquid antibacterial soap and swipe with alcohol. Do the same to the area to be plucked.

Use the best grade tweezers you can afford. I have several patients who have requested that I order a special set of surgical tweezers for them. They are available through Milltex Surgical Instruments, Lake Success, New York. Ask for SWISS CILIA FORCEPS (516-349-0001).

If your skin is very sensitive, place an ice cube on the skin to numb the area before tweezing.

Tweeze as close to the base of the hair as possible without damaging the skin.

EPILATING

This is a mechanical form of tweezing, and most people find it painful and awkward. The devices are made of a rotating coiled spring that traps the hair and pulls it. The possibility of damaging or irritating your skin looms large and, in my opinion, is simply not worth it.

THREADING

Threading involves twisting cotton thread around the hair, catching it and removing it at the follicle level. This technique originated in India, but you can find salons that offer threading in major cities. It offers few benefits over waxing except to people who are allergic to it.

WAXING

This method has been used for centuries. It is a relatively quick way to remove unwanted hair for three to eight weeks. The pain involved is intense but brief. Warm wax is applied to the skin. A cheesecloth is applied over the area and then rapidly removed, pulling hair out by the roots. Your operator's skill and experience will have a direct impact on pain and precision. In order for waxing to be effective, the hair you are removing must be sufficiently long to be pulled out. Hair should be at least one-sixteenth of an inch for optimal removal. Hair that is not excessively thick yields the best results.

Although beauty magazines tout the benefits of various waxes, such as beeswax with pine essence and green wax made with resin, these added ingredients do not affect the ultimate outcome and may actually be irritating or allergenic for certain sensitive individuals. Even careful waxing can result in redness and/or minor swelling. Use only cool water and no soap, deodorant or powder for twenty-four to forty-eight hours after waxing.

Another type of waxing, cold waxing, eliminates the need for heat but is usually more expensive. There is no distinct advantage of cold over hot waxing.

DEPILATORY CREAMS

Most commercial depilatory products contain thioglycolate which reduces the strength of hair fibers by breaking the bonds between the hair and the hair shaft. Thioglycolate causes relatively less irritation to the skin compared to an ingredient such as sodium hydroxide (lye). Stick with brand-name products such as NAIR, NEET and SALLY HANSEN and never leave depilatory cream on your skin for more than ten minutes.

Slower regrowth and a pain-free experience are the main advantages of depilatory creams and lotions. In some cases, however, especially when depilatories are used on the face, irritation can occur. The best places on the body to use depilatories are the bikini line, upper thigh and legs. Dark and/or coarse hair is more resistant to removal by depilatories than light, fine hair.

Men who have difficulty with ingrown beard hair (pseudofolliculitis barbae), most commonly found among African Americans, should use products containing barium sulfide. Do not use these more than every other day and never apply them on abraded or irritated skin.

HOW TO USE DEPILATORIES

Soak the skin in warm water for five minutes before applying cream. Keep the cream on for the maximum time allotted in the directions, and never use depilatories on broken skin.

Remove the cream with a wet washcloth using light pressure.

Wipe in the opposite direction of the growth. When removing coarser hair (such as from the bikini line), remember to cover all the hair with the depilatory cream so that the underlying skin is not visible.

ELECTROLYSIS

This technique was discovered by an American physician in 1875 and was soon thereafter adopted by nonphysician technicians. It is now performed more often in the United States than anywhere else in the world.

Electrolysis is defined as the removal of hair by the delivery of an electric current to the root by means of a needle.

While electrolysis offers a potentially permanent method of hair removal, the process can be painful and time consuming. Because only hair that is in the active phase of growth is permanently destroyed, repeat visits are often needed. Regrowth can range from 10 to 50 percent and depends upon the skill of the operator.

Shaving several days prior to your electrolysis appointment will ensure that only active hairs will be removed. The bikini line, underarms and any area that tends to develop ingrown hairs are recommended sites for electrolysis.

Risks of electrolysis, including scarring and transmission of bacteria, can be greatly reduced by choosing a well-trained electrologist. Lucy Peters International is a reputable national chain of electrolysis centers that provides dependable, sanitary hair removal. Contact your State Board of Professional Licensures or the State Department of Health if you have concerns about the qualifications of your electrologist.

West Virginia is the only state to restrict electrology to physicians and physician assistants. Twenty-three states do not require licensing of electrologists.

The cost can run $75 to $100 per hour, and in general, twenty-five to one hundred hairs can be removed per sitting.

People with bacterial endocarditis, heart valve surgery, cardiac pacemakers or joint prostheses should not undergo electrolysis. Patients prone to scarring or pigment disorders should consult their dermatologist before undergoing electrolysis.

"Electronic tweezers" and other gadgets advertised in the back of magazines and on infomercials will not provide permanent hair removal.

LASER HAIR REMOVAL

Lasers allow for the removal of large areas of unwanted excess hair with less discomfort and fewer complications than electrolysis. Lasers specifically select pigment-containing hair. The noninvasive nature of the laser, which requires no needles, reduces the risk of scarring. Like electrolysis, however, multiple treatments may be needed because hairs must be in the active phase of growth in order for them to be permanently removed. In many cases, regrowth is slower and hair is finer and lighter in color.

The best candidates for laser hair removal are people with light skin and dark hair. The darker your skin color, the more painful the procedure because pigment within the hair follicle and, incidentally, the skin are targeted by the laser beam.

There are many types of lasers, all of which are in an ongoing state of evolution and improvement. One of the most effective lasers is the Alexandrite model. It is wise to choose a technician who was trained by a medical doctor.

Nails

The basic functions of nails are to protect our fingers, help us grasp objects, increase manual dexterity and facilitate fine touch. We also rely on nails to scratch an itch.

Keeping nails healthy-looking and groomed enhances your overall appearance. Whether you choose to keep your nails long or short, with or without polish, your daily nail care routine should include gentle consistent attention.

BASIC ANATOMY

There are seven basic parts of a normal nail.

1   The proximal nail fold, which is the skin at the base of the nail. This includes the cuticles.

2   The lateral nail fold, which is the skin on either side of the nail.

3   The matrix, which is the growth portion of the nail. You can't see most of the matrix.

4   The lunula, that whitish half-moon area at the bottom of the nail, usually on your thumb.

5   The nail plate, the largest structure of the nail that you actually can see. It's usually pink because it interfaces with many blood vessels.

6   The nail bed, which is hidden by the nail plate.

7   Hyponychium, which is the skin at the tip of the nail. It is usually not visible unless you cut down the nail or pull it back.

Nails grow continuously, unlike your hair which has a resting phase. It takes about six months for a finger-nail to grow out completely, and twelve to eighteen months for a toenail. Nails are very porous, absorbing water and moisture more readily than skin.

Your nails provide a physical diary of the state of your health. Internal disorders—including thyroid dys-function, emphysema and anemia—manifest them-selves on your nails. Some of the more common nail manifestations include:

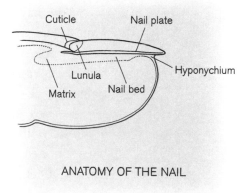

ANATOMY OF THE NAIL

Pitting. Small pitted indentations on the nail can be a symptom of psoriasis. Pitting can also be found in people with lupus, eczema and sar-coidosis.

Clubbing. A swollen spadelike shape at the end of the nail called clubbing is often caused by heart and lung disease. When it is painful, it may suggest lung cancer.

Yellow-nail syndrome. Yellowish nails that grow slowly and in which the lunula and cuticle are absent. The nails are also thickened. This condition is associated with respiratory infections.

Bands of darkened color. Any change in the color of your nail such as darkened bands from the top to the bottom of the nail should be brought to the attention of a dermatologist since this may be a sign of melanoma.

DAILY NAIL CARE

Moisturize your nails as you would your skin. Hand cream or body lotion works well, especially any product that contains alpha hydroxy acids. If your hands and nails are very dry, look for a product that contains urea or lactic acid such as CARMOL 20 EXTRA STRENGTH CREAM or LAC HYDRIN 12 LOTION.

A good and very inexpensive nail moisturizer can be found in your cupboard—vegetable oil. Dab your nails with safflower, corn or olive oil, and massage in gently. The great thing about cooking oil is its absolute purity—no additives, fragrances or other ingredients—and it really works as well as any commercial product.

Trim any excess skin around your nails with small, sharp scissors. Excessively dry nails can lead to hangnails, especially if you have a tendency to bite or pick your nails and the surrounding skin. Don't pull the skin or dig into it. Any trauma to this part of the nail invites infection, not to mention a very unsightly nail.

Remove dirt gently. If there is dirt or debris under the nail, remove it carefully after your shower when the skin and material under the nail have softened. If that doesn't do it, soak your hands in warm water with a tiny bit of baby shampoo and then remove the debris with a moist paper towel or cotton swab. Wooden sticks designed for nail care, sometimes called orange sticks, can be used under the paper towel or swab for difficult-to-reach areas. If you can't remove the dirt after a few tries, quit and try again another day. Digging out dirt when your skin is very dry may lead to injuring the nail and surrounding skin.

After cleaning the nail, shape it with an emery board. A rule of thumb is to shape your nails in the approximate shape of the bottom half. Clip nails with a sharp, clean nail clipper across the top of the nail. Do not cut into the sides of the nail because this can lead to ingrown nails or infection. Injuring the matrix, which is under the cuticle, will cause nails to grow out in a misshapen form.

Keeping your nails covered with either a clear or colored nail enamel can protect them from tearing as well as shield them from drying chemicals. If you have soft nails, protect them with a liquid nail hardener.

Recommended Products
Sally Hansen One Coat Instant Strength
Barielle's Clearly Noticeable Nail Thickener

Use these products alone or before applying a colored enamel. Avoid any nail bases or hardener with formaldehyde since this ingredient can cause nail injury and allergic reactions.

Keep your nails a medium to short length to avoid splitting and breakage, and avoid immersing your hands in water or strong detergent solutions. Wear rubber gloves when possible during cleaning.

In general, nail polish doesn't cause allergic reactions to the nail itself. Certain individuals, however, may develop a reaction (dermatitis) when they scratch their skin or rub their eyes, causing the polish to come in contact with these areas. This allergic reaction occurs when the nail polish hasn't fully dried.

When you want to remove the polish, look for acetone-free nail polish removers, especially ones that contain an emollient such as lanolin or a synthetic oil. Regardless of what type of polish remover you use, it's wise to remove polish no more than once a week, preferably only once every two weeks, to reduce dryness. When removing nail polish, use a cotton ball soaked in polish remover and apply it from the cuticle to the tip. Don't pick off nail polish because you run the risk of removing a layer of nail in the process.

MANICURES
There are eight steps to a good manicure. You can do it at home or treat yourself to a professional manicure.

1   Remove nail polish and allow nails to air dry.
2   Soak your fingers in warm soapy water for five minutes. Add a drop of mineral or olive oil to the water for extra moisturizing. Gently dry with a soft cotton cloth and then gently massage a moisturizing cream into the nail. Rinse and remove excess water and cream.
3   File your nails with an emery board, using a gentle motion in one direction. Use a coarser emery board for shaping and a lighter

board to finish. You should file the nail straight at the sides, being careful not to file the sides in a severe slant.

4 Apply a moisturizer to the cuticles. Remove dirt from the nails with an orange stick covered with a small piece of cotton. Push the cuticles back with a soft towel.

5 Trim the cuticles with a cuticle pusher or cutter. Don't cut too close to the base because this can lead to red swollen cuticles.

6 Apply a base coat in smooth, even strokes.

7 Apply nail polish. Use one steady brush stroke down the center and then do the sides. If your nails are long enough, dab some polish on the underside of the nail for a longer lasting manicure.

8 Apply a clear top coat.

NAIL EXTENDERS

Frustrated by short, weak nails, some women turn to fakes. These products pose a risk of allergic reactions from the adhesive materials that attach them to the natural nail. Sculptured nails are very popular because they can be made to the exact size and shape of your natural nails. The most common type of artificial nails are made of acrylic material and applied over the entire natural nail. Nail wraps, a type of sculptured nail, are made of paper, linen or other material and then are attached with glue. False "tips" can be applied to the sculptured nail to make it look even longer. Check with your manicurist to be sure she is not using Methyl Methacrylate (MMA), a toxic adhesive that was banned twenty-five years ago, but has recently shown up in some salons.

The biggest problem with sculptured nails is what they do to your own nails. Continually wearing artificial nails has been associated with in-fections and misshapen nails.

Never wear sculptured nails for more than three consecutive months. Give yourself a one-month break between applications of sculp-tured nails.

Trauma or application of acrylic artificial nails may cause separation of the nail from the nail bed (onycholysis). This condition permits entry of bacteria or, more commonly, fungus. Fungus may also invade the gap between a fingernail and an artificial nail. These problems can often be traced back to the manicurist. Many states do not require any special license or training for a person to be able to apply artificial nails. Poorly sterilized equipment or careless application of the glue create problems for your nails.

COMMON NAIL PROBLEMS

Severe vitamin deficiencies can cause dryness, brittleness or ridges in the nails. Fortunately, everyday foods such as cauliflower, lentils and peanuts provide the vitamins we need for healthy nails.

For many years gelatin was touted as a cure-all for problem nails. We now know that gelatin doesn't do anything for nails. A well-balanced diet is generally adequate to keep your nails healthy. Biotin, a supplement, has been shown to improve nail thickness and the underlying cell arrangement of the dorsal nail surface. Experts recommend 60 micrograms (mcg) per day.

REMEDIES FOR COMMON NAIL DISORDERS

● *Brittle, cracked nails* are most likely the result of external abuse rather than diet. A recent study showed that 50 percent of women who worked with water suffered from brittle nails. To combat this problem, I recommend greasy emollients. Look for products that contain petroleum, lanolin or mineral oil and protein.

● *Discolored nails* can be cleaned with one part lemon juice and one part water. Soak for no more than three minutes and follow up immediately with a moisturizing cream.

● *Longitudinal ridges,* a normal occurrence especially among older persons, can be treated with gentle buffing every three weeks. Be aware that nail growth slows down during colder weather and with increasing age.

● *Paronychia,* a very common nail infection characterized by redness, swelling, sometimes pus on the side of the nail. Paronychia can be caused by trauma and subsequent infection from bacteria, fungi or yeast. Exposures to water and chemicals are also culprits. For home treatment, use hot compresses or soak your finger in hot water. If the condition does not improve, see your dermatologist.

● *Onychomycosis* is a common condition caused by a fungal infection. It can affect both fingernails and toenails. Symptoms include nails that are thickened, horizontally split and marked by a yellow, green or white discoloration. When the nail fungus becomes serious, it is more than a cosmetic problem. Onychomycosis can interfere with many everyday tasks. Effective systemic treatments include SPORONOX and LAMISIL, available by prescription.

TO AVOID TOENAIL FUNGUS

● Make sure to dry your feet and toenails thoroughly. If possible, blow-dry your feet on a cool setting.
● Wear wool or wool and acrylic blend socks. Take an extra pair of clean socks with you, and change your socks during the day, especially if your feet become wet from sweat or damp weather. It feels great to change soggy socks!
● Wear comfortable, breathable shoes. Leather or other natural materials are best. Shoes should be "broad ended," in other words, no pointy toes.
● Wear flip flops or "shower shoes" when you are at the gym or in any public shower.
● Dust your feet with an antifungal foot powder.
● Keep your toenails groomed and short. This reduces the chance that the nail will break or bend, allowing unwanted materials inside. Cut across the nail and not down into it.
● Get rid of any old shoes that may be serving as a reservoir of infection.
● Keep your eyes on your feet and seek attention promptly if you suspect another outbreak.
● Tell family members to check their feet.

According to James A. Duke, Ph.D., author of *The Green Pharmacy,* a combination of antifungal herbal remedies, both external and internal, may provide relief from fungus. Try drinking chamomile or lemongrass tea or applying the used, cool tea bags directly to the nail. Be careful, however, to air dry your feet after applying the tea bags. Eating garlic is also recommended because garlic is known to have strong antifungal properties. To fight athlete's foot, Dr. Duke recommends soaking the foot in a basin of warm water with crushed garlic bulbs and a little rubbing alcohol.

GENERAL CARE FOR YOUR HANDS

A cruel and well-known irony: The parts of our bodies which people notice most are those that tend to be exposed to the sun—our eyes, our face and our hands. Another irony: Hands derive part of their beauty from their delicate nature, and in dermatology, delicacy equals thin and fragile skin. A younger hand tends to have more subcutaneous fat and appears plumper than an older hand, which often is draped in paper-thin skin out of which veins bulge and bones are more noticeable. The other "aging" giveaway of hands are so-called liver spots.

If you are considering any kind of rejuvenation treatment either at home or from a professional, don't forget your hands. Having said that, I would like to take a step back and tell you what you must never do. Sclerotherapy, a treatment usually employed on the legs to reduce varicose or spider veins, is now offered for the hands. This is a dangerous and silly thing to do because the veins on your hands may someday save your life. You should never compromise their integrity for the sake of looks. Sclerotherapy actually shrinks or collapses veins. Hand veins can provide important access for intravenous medication in an emergency situation. You want thick, plump, available veins on your hands when medical personnel look for a place to start an IV.

There are other, safer ways to have younger-looking hands. First of all, use sunscreen on them. Wear gloves as much as possible. They can be quite fashionable throughout the spring. Invest in a few lightweight cotton pairs that coordinate with your coats and jackets. If people think you're eccentric, so what? You'll end up with pretty hands.

Keep your hands well moisturized. Soft hands are less likely to suffer from nicks and paper cuts. Keep an extra tube of hand cream in your desk drawer.

At night, use an alpha hydroxy acid moisturizer mixed with a little body moisturizer. Cover your hands with a pair of cotton gloves or gym socks before going to sleep. Doing this once or twice a week will result in smoother-looking hands.

Try using a bit of lemon juice on your hands to see if it will lighten brown spots. If that fails, continue to use alpha hydroxy acid products diligently. When you feel you have reached the maximum benefit of these products, you may want to see a dermatologist who can offer stronger AHA peels or Retin-A. You can also inquire about fillers such as fat transplantation for your hands if they appear bony. In this procedure, fat from another part of your body (buttocks, thighs) is removed and injected into the hands. While this treatment lasts only about four to eight months, it is relatively safe and can create an improved appearance.

Some handy hand-care products

AQUAPHOR, which is great for very dry skin and the cuticle area, and is wonderful for paper cuts and other minor abrasions

NEUTROGENA HAND CREAM NORWEGIAN FORMULA, UNSCENTED

KIEHL'S VERY UNUSUALLY RICH BUT NOT GREASY AT ALL HAND CREAM WITH SUNSCREEN SPF 8 (that's really the name of it)

CURÉL SOOTHING HANDS LOTION (great if you wash your hands often)

Now that you know how to wash your face and take care of your nails, hands and hair, we can start talking about what other steps you can take to improve the way you look. In the chapters that follow, I will be providing you with a customized blueprint for your Skin Profile. With this background you can change your daily routine into a personalized approach to better and younger looking skin.

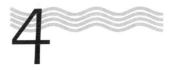

4

Your Skin Profile: Analyzing the "Why" of Your Skin

We have heard it many times before—dry skin, oily skin and combination skin. Three neat categories aimed at selling products to consumers eager for a quick dermatological analysis—but, in my opinion, very inadequate to cover subtle and important variations, particularly among women.

Some of my patients don't know whether their skin tends to be oily or dry. Others know which category they fall into but either aren't sure how to care for their skin or are dissatisfied with the results of their regimen. Women with oily skin tend to scrub with soap and avoid anything with oil, but they still break out with pimples and have shiny skin. Women with dry skin tend to purchase dozens of moisturizers but suffer from a parched, older look. Those with combination skin purchase all kinds of products—exfoliaters, toners, moisturizers and soaps—but still can't seem to find the right balance. When one of my patients described her skin care routine, it sounded like a full-time job. Another became so frustrated that he quit taking care of his skin altogether—and it showed.

In order to help these men and women, I began to analyze their skin difficulties using categories other than the standard oily, dry and combination. I realized that the three traditional skin types characterized skin but did not define the mechanisms and reactions that caused the problems. They just described a symptom. It would be like telling a patient that something was wrong with his leg but not explaining whether it was a muscle spasm, a circulation problem or an infection.

After hundreds of discussions with all different types of patients, I discovered that the most important question was not "What type of skin do you have?" but *"Why* is your skin behaving this way?" Heredity? Lifestyle? Stress? Diet? Too little sleep? Too much alcohol? The wrong skin care? I also wanted to know *when* their skin acted up. Was the change dependent on the weather? Was it linked to emotional troubles or allergy season? When we talked about these issues, a pattern emerged; more important, we identified a way to handle problems with a specific but simple treatment plan.

Once you understand the *why* and *when* of your skin, you will have the key to better care and healthier, more beautiful skin.

Let's review the dry, oil and combination skin types and how this categorization falls short. Then I will introduce you to another perspective—the Skin Profile.

Dry skin looks older than it should. It also feels awful—itchy, flaky and irritated. Skin is continually losing moisture to the atmosphere, especially when humidity is low, such as during winter months. When water is lost faster than it can be replaced from underlying tissue, the outer layer dries out. For the skin to look normal and healthy, the water content of the stratum corneum must be above 10 percent.

In biological terms, dry skin may be the result of a slowdown in the way the skin sheds, causing its outermost layer to become abnormally thick and stiff, inclined to flake or crack. In dry skin the amount of fatty molecules (lipids) within the skin that holds the top layer of cells together is decreased. Lipids also create a barrier to trap and prevent excessive water loss. When these lipids can't perform their job, cells collect on the outermost layer—the layer that you and everyone else sees. Instead of sloughing off, the cells form hard patches that crack and peel. Microscopic studies show that dry skin has a thick, cracked and disorganized stratum corneum.

Skin can be dry for many reasons, ranging from the way we wash to the condition of our thyroid gland, to the changes that come with aging.

If one of your parents had dry skin, you may have a genetic predisposition toward it. If you have dry skin, it is important to evaluate why your skin is the way it is.

For example, in some situations, especially among older persons, a standard moisturizer may not adequately treat dry skin if the roughness is caused by the failure of cells to slough off properly. Products containing alpha hydroxy acid may provide more relief than a moisturizer in that case.

In some situations, people with *oily skin* may actually be washing excessively. They may have overactive oil (sebaceous) glands, possibly due to stress, hormonal disorders or genetics.

In your teens and twenties, oily skin may have seemed like a curse as you continually had to powder your nose and blot your face to keep the shine down. You may also have had lots of acne breakouts. As you got older, however, your tendency to be oily became a blessing. People with oily skin tend to have smoother, less wrinkled skin than people with dry skin.

Caring for oily skin presents a challenge because it is subject to acne breakouts. When acne persists beyond a person's teens and twenties, one is faced with fighting both aging skin and blemishes, a difficult task.

The term *combination skin,* developed by cosmetic companies, not dermatologists, refers to skin that is oily in the center of the face (nose, forehead) and dry on the periphery. According to so-called beauty experts, persons with combination skin may break out more often on the oily parts while other areas of their face need more moisture. Combination skin describes obvious physical characteristics, but the underlying cause of the problem is not addressed. No cosmetic foundation has been developed that can supply the proper amount of moisturizing to dry areas while absorbing oil from other areas.

Uncovering the reason for overabundant oil production is the first step toward improving combination skin; and the reason for the dryness must be determined as well. In many cases the misuse of various cosmetic products creates combination skin in the first place. Aggressive cleaning with irritating ingredients can stimulate oil production in the central portion of the face and dry out the skin on the periphery. No wonder, therefore, that so many people find their skin both dry and oily.

Department Store Skin Analysis

Have you ever had your skin analyzed in a department store? It's common for many cosmetic companies to offer this service.

Bright lights, shiny glass countertops, exotic feminine fragrances, elegant jars and bottles, and beautiful women with lab coats—an exciting, sometimes irresistible setting. Always on the first floor, it's hard to miss. And unlike the clerks at the hosiery counter, the sales force is eager to serve you, sometimes leaping from a promotional display to grab your attention. "May I help you?" "Free gift with purchase today!" "Would you like your skin analyzed?" But what are you really getting when you have your skin examined in a department store?

You'll probably end up with very little valuable information. For one thing, you won't be asked to take your clothes off in the middle of Macy's! Because of that, 95 percent of your skin goes ignored. Overlooking body, arm and leg skin is like buying a car based on the condition of the headlights. The skin on the area below your neck reveals important information. Your inherent skin color and texture show up on areas not generally exposed to the sun, such as the inside of your forearm and your buttocks. Without comparing these two areas of skin, the analysis misses an important clue about what type of sunscreen you need. Without the comparison between face and body skin, it's hard to say how much damage has already been done and whether it is sun related or purely chronological.

Consider also that a department store analysis usually takes about three or four minutes. Their mission is to analyze and sell quickly. They can't delve into lifestyle, family history and personal habits. Even if they did, you might not be willing to discuss personal issues with a cosmetic salesperson in front of other people. But that kind of information is critical. A thirty-two-year-old actress, for example, has concerns that are very different from those of a twenty-six-year-old stay-at-home mother. And what about your willingness or ability to comply with beauty routines? Some people have only a limited amount of time for skin care. Others wear lots of makeup and spend hours in front of the mirror.

Additionally, information about what prescription and nonprescription drugs you are taking could explain why a skin condition exists in the first place. Smearing more creams and lotions on a drug-related skin condition will do nothing but waste your money and possibly exacerbate the problem you wanted relieved.

Finally, a department store skin assessment is biased by the motive of the salesperson—who wants to sell you something! Her opinion will be influenced by the products she can get you to buy. I have spoken to many women who feel intimidated into buying something even when they didn't need it or couldn't afford it.

Of course, other women enjoy the department store experience. I'm not suggesting that they should not have a little fun and pick up a few new products to enjoy. My message is that you should go in with your eyes open. You should know a lot about your skin. You should be able to ask the right questions and obtain answers. A bit of healthy skepticism can be quite empowering.

The Skin Profile Questionnaire

Your skin is as complicated as you are. It changes as the years go by or sometimes as seasons and weather challenge its delicate nature. It reacts to insults. It needs attention. Based on these ideas, I have devised a series of questions that will help you determine your Skin Profile. The answers to the questions below will provide you with a truly meaningful assessment of what you need for your skin. The Skin Profile questionnaire uncovers important physiological and psychological issues that affect your skin.

As stated earlier, the three traditional skin types of dry, oily and combination can be a starting point, and they will be discussed in the context of these skin profiles.

Your Skin Profile will be easy to identify. You will find yourself saying "That's me" with great conviction to one specific category. You will also learn a lot about what you've been doing right and wrong for your skin.

Consider the following Skin Profile questions.

HORMONALLY REACTIVE SKIN

- Do you break out before your period?
- Is your face relatively clear at other times of the month?
- Do you tend to break out on your jawline or neck?
- Are your pimples painful and/or deep?
- Have you noticed dark patches of skin on your face after sun exposure?
- Do you use oral contraceptives? Have you noticed an improvement or worsening in your skin since using oral contraceptives?
- Are you or could you be pregnant? Have you noticed any skin changes during pregnancy for better or worse?
- Have you experienced missed menstrual periods without being pregnant?
- Have you developed facial hair, a deeper voice, or other masculine features?
- Have you ever been diagnosed with polycystic ovary disease or adrenal hyperplasia?
- Are you menopausal or perimenopausal?
- Have you noticed any changes in your skin since you became menopausal such as thinner, drier skin or a chronic problem with blemishes?
- Are you undergoing estrogen replacement therapy (ERT)?

STRESS-REACTIVE SKIN

- How stressful is your life, on a scale of 1 to 10 with 10 being the highest level of stress?
- Do you suffer from any illness such as high blood pressure, ulcers or heart disease that has been attributed in some part to stress?
- Does your skin have a tendency to break out during times of stress?
- Do you suffer from psoriasis, eczema or generalized itchiness and/or hives notice that the condition worsens when you are feeling stressed?
- Have you ever created or aggravated a skin condition by touching or picking your skin?

- Does your occupation require you to travel?
- Do you fly on airplanes more than four times a month?
- Do you engage in any stress-reducing techniques such as exercise, meditation, hobbies, volunteering, and so forth?

ENVIRONMENTALLY SENSITIVE SKIN

- Do you have a personal history or a family history of eczema, asthma or hay fever?
- Do you have any type of allergies?
- Has your skin ever been affected by products or ingredients such as glue, dyes or rubber gloves?
- Have you ever had a skin reaction to perfumes, cologne, soaps, creams or other products that you used on your face or body?
- Do you have an exaggerated response to bug bites or stings?
- Are you taking any of the following drugs?
  Antibiotics such as penicillin or tetracycline
  Nonsteroidal anti-inflammatories such as aspirin, or ibuprofen
  such as NUPRIN, ALEVE, MOTRIN or NAPROSYN
  Diuretics such as hydrochlorothiazide
  Sulfa drugs such as BACTRIM
  Oral contraceptives
- Do you have any of the following medical conditions?
  Polymorphous light eruption
  Lupus erythematosus
  Rosacea

OVEREXPOSED SKIN

- Are your eyes blue?
- Is your hair red or blond?
- Is the skin on your inner arms pale white?
- Do you have brown spots or irregular areas of color on your skin?
- Do you have freckles?
- Do you have a history of skin cancer?
- Does anyone in your immediate family have a history of skin cancer?
- Did you spend a lot of time outdoors as a child or teenager?

- Do you sunbathe?
- Is the condition of your facial skin more wrinkled and/or more tanned than other parts of your body that have not been exposed to the sun?

LIFESTYLE ANALYSIS

- How much time can you spend every day caring for your skin?
  Ten minutes or less
  Ten to twenty minutes
  More than twenty minutes
- Do you live in an area of the country with high levels of pollution?
- Do you wear foundation every day or almost every day?
- Do you wear sunscreen on your face with an SPF of 15 or greater on a regular basis?
- Have you considered plastic surgery to correct what you consider signs of aging?

These are the types of questions I ask my patients in order to determine their Skin Profile. The answers reveal much about what's making their skin look and feel bad. I ask even more specific questions depending on what I learn about the patient. For example, I recently saw a local newscaster who had a mysterious rash on his leg. After seeing an internist who was concerned that he might have lupus, an autoimmune disease, he came to my office. I asked this man many questions, but no single answer gave me a clue. Just as he was getting ready to leave, I inquired whether he ever used a space heater. He said he did. The television studio where he worked on the early morning shift was quite cold, so he put a heater under his anchor desk. That was the information I needed. I diagnosed him with a disorder called erythema ab igne caused by chronic heating of the skin, and his problem was solved. The condition is easily treated by avoiding exposure of the skin to direct heat.

My recommendation is that you reevaluate your Skin Profile every six months or so to determine if it has changed and to adjust your skin care regimen accordingly.

Think carefully about these questions and your answers to them. They are not meant to be judgmental. They are meant to provide you with insight about the dynamic nature of your skin and its reaction to your emotions, external irritants and other factors.

Five Skin Profiles

I have devised a treatment plan for five Skin Profiles, which I will discuss in the following chapters.

1 Hormonally Reactive
2 Stress Reactive
3 Environmentally Sensitive
4 Overexposed
5 Hearty

If you found that the most relevant questions related to your menstrual cycle or other hormonal changes, you may have Hormonally Reactive Skin.

If you found that the stress-related issues caused your skin trouble, your skin is Stress Reactive.

As their names imply, Hormonally Reactive and Stress-Reactive Skin respond to changes within your body. These changes result from chemicals and hormones circulating within your bloodstream that show up on your skin. Reactive skin types can be oily, dry, combination or even "normal."

If your skin reacts most strongly to outside elements such as heat, weather changes, insect bites, irritating fabrics, soaps, creams or cosmetics, your skin is Environmentally Sensitive. Your skin responds in an exaggerated fashion to contact with the outside world.

Did you find after reviewing the questions that your skin was not truly reactive or sensitive? Instead, your concerns revolved around the aged appearance of your skin—lines, furrows, brown spots, and rough texture. Most likely, your skin profile is Overexposed. It has been damaged by the environment, specifically ultraviolet radiation. In some cases Overexposed skin has also been damaged by harsh products. This type of skin has begun to show signs of photoaging in the form of wrinkles, dark spots and spider veins. This category of skin is neither too sensitive nor reactive but instead has photo-age-related problems.

A few fortunate people may find that none of the questions apply to them. Their skin may not show any sensitivity to hormones, stress or the environment. Either through sun avoidance or because of good genes, or both, your skin may not be showing any signs of premature aging. If this sounds like you, the category of Hearty Skin fits.

Golden Rules for All Five Skin Types

Some rules hold true for all skin types. They are simple and straightforward, and will produce lasting results if you follow them.

1 Use sunscreen. It's a must for everyone. As of this date, there is no single sunscreen ingredient that completely protects against the entire spectrum of both UVA and UVB radiation. Some sunscreen labels that read "broad spectrum" are misleading because manufacturers can make this claim even if their product provides just a little UVB protection or a little UVA protection. The so-called broad spectrum sunscreens should be called "partial dual protection." Still, broad spectrum sunscreens are the best products available. A sunscreen with an SPF of 15 should be used on the face every day.

2 Be skeptical of products that promise everything. Do not be seduced by the names of products. You really can't get a face-lift in a bottle. Catchy buzzwords such as "face-lift," "firming," "youth," and so forth, are used for products that may work well at diminishing the appearance of wrinkles or lightening dark spots, but they are not going to pull your skin back to where it was when you were younger. You may still wish to buy the product, but be aware of inflated promises.

3 Introduce your skin to acids. I am a big fan of alpha hydroxy and beta hydroxy acids. Used correctly, they can decrease acne breakouts, smooth lines, soften the texture of your skin and lighten brown spots. Used incorrectly, however, they can be irritating and cause your skin to become blotchy. Many people start using an AHA or BHA only to stop be-

cause of unpleasant side effects. Refer to specific recommendations throughout this book for an AHA product that is best suited for you.

4 See a dermatologist if you have a changing skin growth. If you have a mole, pimple or growth of any kind on your body that is changing in size, shape or color, or is not healing, seek the advice of a dermatologist. Do not try to treat it or remove it yourself. Be aware of signs such as bleeding or itching.

5 Don't bother with separate creams for different parts of your face. Cosmetic companies make a lot of money by selling you a variety of products for different parts of the body, such as eye cream, neck cream, bust cream and leg cream. The major ingredients in these products vary very little. If you have an effective face cream, just apply a little extra of it to your eyes for more moisture. To save money, use large pump bottles of standard drugstore moisturizers for your body. Some people enjoy foot creams with peppermint or menthol for their cooling sensation. You can apply a bit of peppermint essential oil to your body cream and turn it into foot cream.

You now have the basic information you need to analyze and understand your skin. The next step is to change the way you care for your skin. This will not complicate your life. In fact, once you recognize the why and how of your skin, your daily skin care routine will be quite simple—and the results will be truly fantastic.

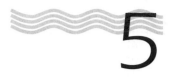

5

Hormonally Reactive Skin

- Do you experience predictable acne flares prior to your period?
- Are you over thirty, but still breaking out with pimples?
- Has your skin changed with the onset of menopause?
- Do you have dark blotches on your cheeks and forehead?

Every system in your body interconnects and reacts with others. Respiration can increase or decrease as the result of emotional responses. Our digestive system slows down or speeds up depending on hormonal, circulatory and mental changes. Likewise, skin is an unerring reflection of internal harmony, strife and conflict.

Hormones rule. At least 130 different kinds of hormones circulate through our body, acting as chemical messengers. It is difficult to name any system or function in our bodies that is not affected by them. Our energy, moods, weight and ability to reproduce are all regulated by hormones. Ancient Greeks identified hormones as an agent that can "excite" or "arouse." At their most basic level, hormones do just that. The signals they send can speed up, slow down, stimulate and even interfere with the function of every organ and cell. We have only begun to appreciate how profoundly hormones affect us both physically and emotionally. Considering the powerful influence of hormones, it should come as no surprise that our skin is subject to their fluctuations. And some people are affected more directly than others.

Hormonal Acne

Acne originates in the pilosebaceous glands that house both hair follicles and oil (sebum) glands. These glands are found in the greatest abundance on the face, scalp, back and chest. When sebum is blocked by accumulated skin cells and cannot exit normally to the skin surface, blackheads develop. The black color is not dirt but rather keratin (dead skin cells) and oil that have been oxidized (exposed to the air). Sebum continues to accumulate beneath the blocked pore. A particular kind of bacteria, called *P. acnes,* normally present within the pore, proliferates as well. This volatile collection of oil and bacteria eventually outgrows the limited space at the base of the follicle and ruptures into the surrounding skin. Inflammation ensues, and a red swollen pimple results. Doctors call red acne bumps "papules" and whitish pus bumps "pustules." Whiteheads are pustules. Many patients have "pustular" acne, inflamed bumps and whiteheads. When the follicle ruptures deep within the skin with severe inflammation, a cyst is formed. This is called "cystic acne." These large, painful pimples have a propensity to form scars.

Although we understand the physical mechanics of acne, the more troublesome question is why our skin overproduces sebum. In some cases, the answer is hormones. If you tend to break out with acne before or during your period, or you notice changes for the better in your skin while using the birth control pill, your skin is hormonally reactive. This type of skin can also react to changes within the body during pregnancy, breastfeeding and menopause.

A predictable premenstrual flare, or blemish, is a hallmark of hormonal acne.

Considerable evidence has linked a type of hormone called androgen with acne in up to 50 percent of affected women. Androgens are generally considered male sex hormones; they are produced in the

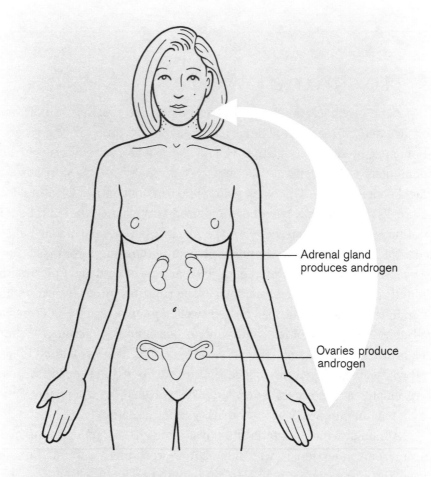

Adrenal gland
produces androgen

Ovaries produce
androgen

HORMONALLY REACTIVE SKIN

Hormonal acne may be caused by the release of androgens from ovaries and
adrenal glands prior to menstruation. Postmenopausal acne may be caused by
decreased levels of estrogen and the relative abundance of androgens. Hormonal
acne is typically seen on the lower face and on the neck.

adrenal glands located on the top of each kidney but also in the ovaries in women.

Fortunately, the majority of women with hormonal acne do not need treatment aimed at lowering androgen levels. Instead they need to follow a skin care plan that correlates with hormonal fluctuations.

For years dermatologists have recognized that specific hormonal disorders affect the skin. Women with severe acne that does not respond to standard treatments may need to undergo hormonal testing to determine if they are suffering from a systemic illness for which their acne is an external manifestation. In rare instances, hormonally based conditions such as polycystic ovary disease or adrenal hyperplasia may be the underlying cause of acne. Excess hair on the upper lip and chin, menstrual irregularities, male-pattern hair loss and obesity are other symptoms of polcystic ovary disease. In adrenal hyperplasia, women develop masculine features such as increased facial hair and deepening of the voice.

In many cases, hormonal problems can be assessed through blood tests. Once the medical condition is treated, the acne responds as well.

But what about the thousands of women who have breakouts around their period but have no detectable hormonal abnormalities? This scenario is much more common. Premenstrual exacerbation of acne is experienced by as many as 60 percent of women, the majority of whom have no known hormonal problems.

This chapter focuses mainly on women whose hormonal levels are normal but who report changes in their skin every month. A possible explanation for this phenomenon is an overproduction of oil triggered by an exaggerated response to normal hormonal fluctuations.

Dawn

Ever since she was a young woman, Dawn had problems with her period—it was either late or altogether absent. Dawn's skin, however, was clear as a teenager. Unlike a lot of her friends, Dawn never got acne.

In her twenties, Dawn became an avid runner—six days a week, seven miles a day. She ran marathons, ate a healthy diet and seemed to be in perfect health. Dawn recalls that she had "great skin" as well. During this time, Dawn's periods stopped.

Although she was not my patient then, I believe Dawn was experiencing exercise-induced amenorrhea—the cessation of menstruation as the result of a very low body fat content.

While jogging one morning, Dawn hurt her knee. The injury sidetracked her running, and after a few months without exercise her period resumed. Along with her period, Dawn began experiencing skin problems for the first time in her life.

"I used to be able to put on any kind of lotion, and my skin wouldn't break out. Now I have to be very careful," she told me.

In addition to acne problems, Dawn noticed that she was developing dark blotchy spots on her face. I diagnosed this condition as melasma, a pigment disorder related to hormones.

"My skin is much worse right before my period," she said.

Dawn is a perfect example of Hormonally Reactive Skin. The changes taking place within her body appear on her skin. By using Retin-A and a mild alpha hydroxy cleanser, Dawn has been able to control her breakouts. She is more aware that she needs to adjust her skin care routine according to monthly cycles.

ADULT-ONSET ACNE

"I thought I'd be over with acne by the time I was twenty-nine!"

"I didn't even have pimples when I was a teenager."

"All of a sudden, my skin is breaking out. I feel like an adolescent even though I'm the mother of two teenagers."

These are the kinds of comments I hear at least once a day from educated, hardworking women. One of the fastest-growing groups of acne patients is women from twenty-five to forty-plus. Acne is distressing at any age, but in adult females it can create a level of self-consciousness that interferes with personal and professional relationships. Indeed, adult-onset acne is a problem uniquely wrought from our westernized, late-twentieth-century, go-go society. As career pressures and family obligations mount, women find breakouts becoming more and more common. According to some experts, acne occurs in about 50 percent of upwardly mobile women.

Individuals with adult-onset acne are in the unenviable position of dealing with pimples and the early signs of aging skin. This is a prime example of how the dry, oily and combination skin categories have become oversimplified and outdated. Who would ever have associated dry skin with acne? But I see patients with dry skin and acne every day.

Adult-onset acne can occur in women with Hormonally Reactive or Stress-Reactive Skin. As a matter of fact, hormonal acne and stress-related acne are various types of adult-onset acne. For this reason, I will discuss both of these problems in this chapter.

One of the most common problems of adult-onset acne is large, deep, painful pimples. For women with Hormonally Reactive Skin, these blemishes erupt before their period. For women with Stress-Reactive Skin, emotional upheaval can stimulate a breakout.

According to one theory, emotional upset causes the adrenal glands to produce cortisone, which in turn causes sebum production from sebaceous glands. Excess oil production combined with a buildup of dead skin cells results in clogged pores, which can evolve into acne. Often these blemishes don't come to a head but remain under the skin.

There is no concrete evidence that acne of any kind is caused by diet or poor hygiene. However, physical manipulation of the skin such as scrubbing or touching the face, certain medications and too much sun have been implicated.

For women with premenstrual syndrome, hormonal changes produce stress, mood swings, food cravings and sometimes depressive symptoms. Their skin can also suffer during this time. In these situations it may be difficult to know whether your skin is Hormonally or Stress Reactive. *The best way to distinguish between the two is to notice whether your skin becomes troublesome not just before your period but at other stressful times at well.*

Stress-related acne is a lot less predictable than hormonally reactive acne. There are no set times when you can expect a breakout. On those occasions when you can anticipate stress, however, such as a job change, important examinations or major events in your life, you should be especially conscientious about your skin care regimen.

Keep a record of when your skin tends to break out. It's a good idea to keep two small skin care or makeup bags handy—one for clear times and one for hormonal flares.

At-Home Care

CLEANSING

The treatment depends on the severity of the condition. When your skin is clear (nonmenstrual and nonstressed), you can use:

EXUVIANCE PURIFYING GEL CLEANSER by Neostrata (609-520-0715)

M.D. FORMULATION OIL-FREE CLEANSER by Allergan, which is available in better beauty salons, or call 800-MDFORMULA

ALPHA HYDROX FOAMING FACE WASH by Neoteric Cosmetics, Inc. (800-55-ALPHA)

Use no more than twice a day, preferably once in the evening to remove makeup, and dirt.

Some people find alpha hydroxy acid products a bit irritating. In that case, I recommend alternating their use with one of the following:

LANCÔME CLARIFIANCE OIL-FREE GEL CLEANSER

NEUTROGENA FRESH FOAMING CLEANSER

BASIS PURE AND SIMPLE EXTRA GENTLE FACIAL CLEANSER

If your skin is very oily, try SEBA NIL SKIN CLEANSER or NEUTROGENA SOAP.

During breakout times, you need to alter your skin program somewhat. Cleanse your face once or twice a day with

NEUTROGENA EXTREMELY GENTLE ACNE FOAM

MURAD ADVANCED ACNE PRONE FORMULA

CLEARASIL MEDICATED DEEP CLEANSER or FOSTEX ACNE CLEANSING CREAM

For oilier skin during breakout times, try FOSTEX 10% WITH BENZOYL PEROXIDE.

Whichever product you use, avoid washing your face too often. Twice a day is adequate. Don't use a washcloth. Instead, wet your face with tepid water and use your fingertips to wash. Vigorous scrubbing can aggravate acne.

When using any cleanser, first wet your face with cool water and then apply the cleanser, being sure to cover the areas where you are apt to break out. Leave it on for a minute, and then splash off thoroughly with tepid water.

MOISTURIZING

If your skin is very oily, you don't need a moisturizer. However, if your skin is dry *and* you still break out, you need to use the right kind of moisturizer. Look at the label of your moisturizer and make sure the first ingredient is a sunscreen. Look for oil-free moisturizers labeled non-comedogenic (won't cause blackheads) and nonacnegenic (won't cause acne). While these labels are not a guarantee that they won't cause you to break out, they are a good starting point.

Apply the moisturizer after cleansing, while your face is still moist but not dripping wet.

For daylight hours, moisturizers with sunscreen are recommended for skin that is dry or normal, such as PHYSICIANS FORMULA SELF-DEFENSE MOISTURIZING LOTION SPF 15 or OIL OF OLAY DAILY UV PROTECTANT LOTION SPF 15.

Allow the moisturizer to soak in for a minute or so before applying foundation or other makeup.

After cleansing your skin at night, treat it with ingredients that will help keep acne at bay. Two good inexpensive night products are POND'S AGE-DEFYING LOTION (8% AHA) and POND'S AGE-DEFYING LOTION FOR DELICATE SKIN (4% AHA). CLINIQUE'S TURNAROUND LOTION contains salicylic acid and is ideal for oily or breakout-prone skin as a night cream. Some of my patients have told me that they apply Turnaround Lotion with a makeup sponge and have found they get a more even application and mild exfoliation effect in the process.

Salicylic acid is one of the best ingredients for treating acne. A salicylic acid product reduces blackheads and inflamed pimples. It is gentler on the skin than alpha hydroxy acid for persons who are particularly sensitive. Salicylic acid with concentrations from .5 percent to 2 percent is recommended.

I have been appalled to see so-called beauty experts claiming that salicylic acid and benzoyl peroxide don't work against acne. They do work if used consistently. Begin to use them a week before you expect to break out. They're easy to find in the drugstore.

For spot treatment and to camouflage pimples, try CLINIQUE'S ANTI-ACNE CONTROL FORMULA or NEUTROGENA ON-THE-SPOT ACNE TREATMENT. Both contain benzoyl peroxide. For a medicated treatment to use in the evening, try ALMAY CLEAR COMPLEXION ACNE POST MEDICATION CREAM WITH SALICYLIC ACID.

SUN PROTECTION

Your skin needs sun protection every day even if it tends to break out. If you choose not to wear moisturizer, you should wear a sunscreen product. Sunblocks should be nonirritating, nonstinging and nonacnegenic. Look for a product that you are comfortable using every day. Compliance and consistency are the keys to keeping skin looking great, and a product that you like ensures compliance.

Gels are water-based and are a good choice for acne-prone skin. Some choices are:
SHADE SUNBLOCK GEL SPF 25 OR 30, CLINIQUE'S CITY BLOCK OIL-FREE DAILY FACE PROTECTOR SPF 15, which has a slight tint, and PRE-SUN ACTIVE CLEARGEL SUNSCREEN 30.

IS MAKEUP TO BLAME?

A lot of my patients think that makeup is a cause of their acne. We now know this occurs only on rare occasions. Cosmetics may aggravate preexisting acne by creating more blackheads (comedones) or a mild form of inflamed hair follicles (folliculitis), but they generally don't start the problem. For the most part, nonacnegenic and noncomedogenic products work very well for people with acne-prone skin. Pomades for the hair are known to cause acne. Other than that, most doctors agree that "acne cosmetica" is overdiagnosed.

ON-THE-SPOT TREATMENT FOR ACNE

For instant emergency care, place an ice cube on deep painful pimples for two minutes to reduce their inflamed appearance. VISINE EYE-DROPS or any eyedrop product that removes red will also cut down on the inflamed appearance of a pimple. MILK OF MAGNESIA or CALAMINE LOTION can also dry up pimples and is best used overnight. If you are good in the kitchen, a tomato puree mash blended with nonfat dry milk paste can be placed on the skin for ten minutes.

Keep in mind that no over-the-counter product can change oil *production*. The correct types of cleansers, makeup and moisturizers can provide a temporary change on the surface of the skin that will prevent your face from looking shiny. Careful use of AHA products and gentle cleansers will prevent breakouts during your period. Going overboard with cleansing agents irritates the skin and can make your acne worse.

Do not try to squeeze the pimple or bring it to a head. Try not to overuse products with ingredients such as tallow, peppermint, witch hazel, menthol and alcohol, which can irritate the skin.

Do not use exfoliaters such as scrubs and loofahs more than once a week, if at all. My patients, regardless of skin type, do well without exfoliaters. If you do use a loofah, be sure it is thoroughly dried out between uses and soaked in a solution of one part bleach to ten parts water every two weeks. Otherwise you run the risk of harboring disease-causing bacteria in the sponge. To be perfectly safe, buy a new loofah once a month.

A simple clean makeup sponge can work as a gentle exfoliater. Use it to apply cleansers or skin cream.

Be gentle to your skin. You may be tempted to think you can "disinfect" your pimples away. This is not the case. Remember, hormones, stress and subsequent oil production, not dirt, are your problem.

Professional Care

SURGERY/ANTIBIOTICS

The majority of people with acne don't see a dermatologist for treatment. There may come a time, however, when breakouts become very troublesome and home remedies aren't clearing things up. At this point, a dermatologist should be consulted. You may need to see the dermatologist only once or twice to get things under control. If your budget permits, see the doctor once a month for gentle acne surgery to remove blackheads and a light alpha hydroxy peel that will keep breakouts at bay.

I employ treatments that cause the fewest side effects and get the best results. The latest research shows that up to 50 percent of the bacteria known to cause acne are resistant to some common antibiotic pills used to treat it such as erythromycin and tetracycline. Resistance can result from overusing these drugs.

My approach for patients with Hormonally Reactive Skin is to prescribe antibiotic pills one week before and/or one week after a period, depending on when breakouts occur. This avoids overuse of oral antibiotics and targets the treatment for times when it is most likely to help. Using antibiotics in this time-targeted way reduces the incidence of side effects such as upset stomach, diarrhea and vaginal yeast infections, and the tendency for some people to sunburn more easily. Rarer side effects include dizziness, lightheadedness and headaches.

Antibiotic solutions, gels and lotions usually do not cause the same side effects as pills but may cause occasional bouts of dry skin. On the downside, they are less effective. The consistent use of a topical acne treatment twice a day is equal to about one-half the strength of an antibiotic pill. When used properly, however, topical antibiotics can effectively treat acne, especially in conjunction with benzoyl peroxide.

Topical acne treatment in a solution formulation is best for those with oily skin. CLEOCIN SOLUTION (available by prescription) comes in a sponge-tip applicator bottle that is both convenient and sanitary. My patients with oilier skin like using ERYCETTE PLEDGETTES (available by prescription), which are tiny towelettes in individual packets saturated with a liquid antibiotic that can be wiped over the face once or twice a day.

For persons with drier skin, lotions work best. CLEOCIN LOTION is usually a good choice, especially if you are over thirty and notice that your skin seems dry even though you break out.

RETIN-A AND BEYOND

Retin-A has received such hype as an antiaging treatment that we often overlook its original and still useful purpose: eliminating acne.

Retin-A is a member of the retinoid class of drugs which are vitamin A derivatives. They fight acne by reducing oil production and sloughing material that can clog pores. A second generation of products containing tretinoin offer fewer side effects and sometimes greater efficacy. There is a low incidence of a temporary exacerbation of acne with any retinoid product. After a few weeks this will clear and your acne will be less troublesome over the long run.

One of the newer products, RETIN-A MICRO, available by prescription, is especially effective for Hormonally Reactive Skin because it provides a slow and sustained release that reduces irritation and may also absorb extra oil in the skin.

Newer Retin-A–like drugs also available by prescription include the following:

AZELEX, a cream that soothes inflammation without overdrying

DIFFERIN, a gel that can be used with benzoyl peroxide and produces less redness than Retin-A

AVITA, which can be applied to the skin with less irritation than Retin-A because it does not penetrate as deeply into the skin

I do not recommend TAZORAC because it tends to be irritating.

These products are available in different strengths and formulations (cream, gel, solution) and can be tailored to your particular level of sensitivity. Always use a sunscreen during the day if you are using these products since your skin may be more prone to sun damage.

I do not recommend Retin-A or any related drug during pregnancy or breast feeding.

Dermatologists can also prescribe the pill form of Retin-A called AC-CUTANE for more serious cases of acne (cystic acne). It is one of the most effective choices for problematic acne that is likely to scar. ACCUTANE has serious side effects, and any individual taking it needs to be carefully monitored by a physician. This drug can affect liver function, increase cholesterol, cause stiff joints and ligaments, and reduce night vision. It is also known to cause birth defects among women who use it during pregnancy. Pregnancies several months subsequent to having discontinued the use of ACCUTANE carry no increased risk for birth defects.

In cases where immediate treatment is needed, I inject very swollen, painful pimples with a solution of diluted cortisone for its anti-inflammatory action. In most cases the blemish will begin to shrink within six hours of treatment. Great for auditions, first dates and prom nights!

THE PILL

Certain types of oral contraceptives can reduce acne, but this must be weighed against the risk of side effects such as blood clots and even stroke. It is always best to avoid using any medication unless it is absolutely necessary. The Food and Drug Administration recently approved the oral contraceptive ORTHO-TRI-CYCLEN as a treatment for acne. The results of hormonal treatments usually take about two months to start working.

You should also be aware that certain types of birth control pills can aggravate acne, including LEVLEN, LEVORA, LO/OVRAL, NORDETTE, OVRAL, OVRETTE, TRI-LEVLEN and TRIPHASIL.

Warning

Antibiotics may interfere with the contraceptive effectiveness of the birth control pill. If you are using oral antibiotics for acne, you should use an alternative form of birth control.

POSTMENOPAUSAL ACNE

One skin condition that may occur during menopause is acne. How many women have this problem is unknown, but I have seen patients with acne who are baffled as to why at their age they would suddenly develop pimples. Postmenopausal acne usually occurs within the first two years of menopause, or even a year or two before menopause, and is generally more common in women with thick, darker skin. Scientists theorize that menopausal acne results from the ovaries failing to produce estrogen but continuing to produce androgens. The acne consists of small, scattered, closed blackheads. Exacerbations are uncommon; rather, the condition "smolders." My preferred method of treatment is with Retin-A because it treats both acne and aging skin.

Other Hormonal Skin Problems

Much of this section has been devoted to acne and hormones. The appearance of acne during the menstrual cycle, however, is not the only way that Hormonally Reactive Skin manifests itself. Many women find that pregnancy and menopause affect the appearance and texture of their skin.

THE TRUTH ABOUT HORMONAL CREAMS

Your skin absorbs many of the materials that are applied to it. This has led some cosmetic companies to create lines of products that supposedly contain hormones in hopes that women will use them to combat postmenopausal symptoms. I do not recommend the use of these products for two reasons. First, if the creams actually do contain hormones such as estrogen and progesterone as they claim, people who use them are taking serious risks with their health. According to the FDA, the estrogen count of an over-the-counter product, whether a drug or a cosmetic, may not exceed 10,000 IU (International Units) per ounce. Furthermore, manufacturers must inform consumers that they should limit the amount of product used to no more than 20,000 IU per month. An advisory panel for the FDA has concluded that there are inadequate data to establish the safety of estrogen-containing products that claim to prevent or treat wrinkles and stimulate hair growth. They also concluded that the products are ineffective.

Using hormones, either in pill form or rubbed on the skin, requires the supervision of a physician who can evaluate the exact amounts needed for an intended result. Second (and more likely), these so-called hormonal creams probably do not contain any hormones at all. If they did contain hormones in any significant amount, the FDA would certainly begin investigating whether the cream was actually a drug and not a cosmetic.

Hormones do affect your skin, but you are stepping into dangerous territory if you intend to change your skin by manipulating your own delicate hormonal balance without consulting a doctor first.

SKIN CHANGES DURING PREGNANCY

Changes in the pigment (color) and vascularity (blood vessels) are the two major skin conditions during pregnancy.

Blotches and hormones: melasma. Besides causing acne, hormones can also affect the pigment of your skin. Flat, darkened patches on the forehead, cheeks and upper lips that appear or worsen after sun exposure are called melasma. In contrast to small liver spots caused by the sun that often take years to develop, melasma develops rather quickly. It has the shape of countries on a map. This pigment disorder does not pose any physical harm but can be quite distressing cosmetically.

True to its hormonal origins, melasma often appears first or worsens during pregnancy (and is sometimes called the "Mask of Pregnancy"). More than 50 percent of pregnant women develop at least some degree of melasma. It can also occur when a woman is using birth control pills. It is almost never seen in men.

While the interplay of skin color changes and the hormones of pregnancy is not entirely understood, we do know that many parts of a woman's skin can and do darken during this time, including the nipples, genitalia and the inner thigh. A vertical line down the center of the abdomen called *linea nigra* may also appear. After delivery, these darkened areas may fade, but usually not to the prepregnancy level.

Not only pregnant women get melasma. Dawn, the patient discussed at the beginning of this chapter, developed the blotchy marks of melasma when her hormones began kicking in after her periods reappeared.

The best way to combat melasma is through prevention. Sunblock is essential. You can choose to wear a foundation with sunblock to both protect and conceal. I recommend:

MAYBELLINE NATURAL DEFENSE MAKEUP SPF 15

PRESCRIPTIVES EXACT COLOR MAKEUP 100% OIL-FREE SPF 15

LANCÔME MAQUIMAT and MAQUILIBRE SPF 15
CLINIQUE CITY BASE COMPACT FOUNDATION SPF 15

Products containing hydroquinone are often recommended by physicians to lighten discolored skin. They are available over the counter and by prescription, depending on the strength. I have become reluctant to recommend hydroquinone because of studies that show long-term exposure can induce mutations in genes. Chemicals that cause genetic mutations may have a cancer risk. Many scientists believe there is no safe level of exposure to a cancer-causing agent. While I realize that discolorations of the skin may be distressing, the risk/benefit ratio in this instance does not justify the use of hydroquinone. Safer ingredients should be substituted. For example, lemon juice may fade spots if used full strength every day. Alpha hydroxy acid, kojic acid and azaleic acid can also lighten pigment. AHA is particularly effective when used with Retin-A. Products that contain hydroquinone and should therefore be avoided include PORCELANA, ESOTERICA, MELANEX, ARTA and EXUVIANCE ESSENTIAL SKIN LIGHTENER.

Other skin changes during pregnancy. Pregnant women may find that they develop tiny growths called skin tags on their neck, underarm and other areas. A by-product of hormonal changes, they present no real harm and will often disappear after pregnancy. Moles can change, becoming darker and increasing in size. Although in most cases this is not dangerous, you should see your dermatologist to have the moles examined.

Vascular skin changes during pregnancy include spider veins on the face and red bumps called hemangiomas. Itchiness is also common. To soothe itchy skin, use SARNA lotion which has been cooled in the refrigerator.

During pregnancy, do not use any type of prescription or over-the-counter drug—oral or topical—without first checking with your doctor.

Gentle cleansing is best during this time. Try:
OIL OF OLAY SENSITIVE SKIN FOAMING WASH (UNSCENTED) or AVEDA PURIFYING GEL CLEANSER. Use a nongreasy moisturizer such as CLINIQUE

MOISTURE SURGE or AVEDA OIL-FREE HYDRADERM.

For sun protection, especially for women who are subject to melasma, try MUSTELA 9 RESPONSE PREGNANCY MASK SPF 15.

A woman with Hormonally Reactive Skin knows very well that her skin is subject to changes from day to day. Hormonal Skin will also change through the years. You may find that after the age of thirty-five, blemishes may become less of a problem. The reduction of the size of sebaceous glands and in certain hormone levels will no doubt play a role in your skin's appearance.

Hormonally Reactive Skin requires close attention and special care. Responding to these demands will work to your advantage over time because this will instill effective skin care habits. You will benefit with a lifetime of clearer, healthier, more radiant skin and an understanding of how your body's inner workings have a powerful influence over the way you look.

6

Stress-Reactive Skin

- Do you or other people notice sudden changes in your skin or hair when you are undergoing big changes (good or bad) in your life?
- Have you experienced acne, itchy rashes, hives or other skin eruptions that seem to come and go depending on your level of stress?
- Do you have a tendency to rub, pick or scratch your face while you are reading, studying or thinking about a problem?

If you answered yes to any of these questions, your skin is Stress Reactive.

In this chapter I will discuss how skin responds to stress and ways to diagnose, treat and cope with these problems. A specific event such as a divorce or the loss of a job can evoke a limited but severe stressful episode. During these times an individual may discover how sensitive his or her skin is to emotional turmoil. Managing underlying psychological problems along with the right skin care often helps to clear things up.

While you may not manifest every one of the skin problems described in this chapter, you may have noticed that anxiety and worry affect the quality of your skin. On a brighter note, your skin is much better behaved when things are going well.

◼ Making the Connection

Have you always been aware of your skin-stress connection? If so, you are a step ahead of the game. It takes some people years to realize that their skin is a "stress scorecard." They may fail to admit or recognize they are even under stress. They can delude themselves into thinking that it's just a "coincidence" that their skin started acting up when they became stressed out. After a while, however, the coincidence starts looking more like cause-and-effect.

If you find it hard to believe that your skin can reflect inner feelings, consider this statement by Grossbart and Sherman in *Skin Deep:*

> *Given the skin's intimate bonds with the nervous system, the role of the mind in skin disease should be small surprise; all the more so when you consider that psychologically as well as physically the skin is your boundary with the world outside, at which every act of love, hate, work and play take place.*

I don't want to oversimplify the reason for any one skin condition. It would be unfair and unwise to say that all your breakouts and skin disorders are linked to your state of mind. That would ignore important competing factors such as heredity, underlying medical diseases, medications, infection and allergic reactions which I will discuss in further detail later in this book.

People with Stress-Reactive Skin are not the only ones who have physical reactions to emotional problems. Digestive disorders, chronic headaches, back pain and sexual dysfunction are manifestations of emotional problems with physical symptoms. Saying that you have Stress-Reactive Skin is by no means a way of labeling yourself neurotic. It's merely a way of helping you understand why your skin behaves the way it does and what you can do to significantly reduce or correct the problems you experience.

In some instances it may be difficult to pinpoint how Stress-

Reactive Skin actually starts. Unsightly and chronic conditions such as psoriasis (red, scaly, inflamed skin) and acne cause embarrassment, worry and self-consciousness, which lead to stress. The stress may cause the skin condition to worsen, and the cycle continues. Throughout this chapter, I will be discussing patients who have experienced this phenomenon. This information will help you keep your stress in check and your skin looking healthy.

■ A Word About Stress

Stress permeates our culture. Some people even find it a necessary evil in order to function or complete a project. Others take a perverse pride in their stress load, be it from overworking, personal problems or financial woes. In my practice I meet people in high-stress careers. They juggle family obligations, health problems, financial worries and a host of other pressures. Living in a big city breeds stress that often goes unnoticed but still erodes peace of mind. Pollution, noise, crowding and aggressive—sometimes hostile—interactions with people can all create urban stress. But individuals in smaller communities will admit that other problems irk them and raise their stress level. No matter where we live, we all must deal with unpleasant situations, upheaval, family problems.

Think about what bothers you. Think about what you can do to relieve your stress load. Consider the times when your skin becomes "upset" even though you don't think you are. Stress-Reactive Skin might actually be telling you how you feel.

Perhaps something is making you angry, anxious or worried, but you are having a difficult time admitting it to yourself. Acknowledge your feelings and don't try to dismiss them as "overreacting." Only you know how uncomfortable or anxiety-provoking a situation makes you feel. The most important aspect of my treatment has been helping patients recognize when they have Stress-Reactive Skin.

Denise

Denise, a highly successful attorney, called me from Madrid on a Sunday afternoon to report that her skin was acting up. The rash on her neck, arms and thighs was becoming worse. I had seen her a week prior to her departure and had been puzzled by the rash. There was no apparent diagnosis. Even her skin biopsy results were nonspecific for any disease.

Denise had been to several dermatologists before I saw her. No one was able to arrive at a diagnosis. Sometimes rashes like the one Denise had don't seem to fall squarely into any one category and may actually arise from or be exacerbated by stress. When I first broached the subject of a possible stress-related problem, Denise dismissed the idea.

On the phone from Madrid, I listened as Denise told me that she would be giving an important presentation in three days, and she expressed concern that she would look awful when she did. This made her even more nervous.

Denise told me she was following all the skin care directions that I had provided at the office visit. Her rushed and shaky voice gave me insight into what could have been causing her skin problems: Denise was under tremendous pressure.

"Denise, maybe you should take some time out for yourself," I suggested. "Slow down."

There was silence, then a hesitant "But, I've got to—"

I gently interrupted. "Perhaps you can stop working a little earlier each day during this business trip. Take a stroll or meditate in one of the beautiful museums or parks."

"I don't have the time," she persisted.

"Half an hour?"

"But what does that have to do with my skin?"

"Everything," I replied. There was a short silence. "Are you touching your face right now?"

"How did you know that?" she said.

"I know that you're worried about the way you look and want to improve your skin. Some people tend to touch their face when that happens."

"Hmm. Well, I guess I can try," she said.

A few weeks after she arrived back in New York City, Denise came to see me. She said that her presentation had gone very well. She had decided to heed my advice and took the time to exercise, stretch and relax a little every day. Her skin had *settled down enough to give her the confidence to do the job. After the presentation, she noticed steady improvement.*

We discussed her problem in depth, and she told me that she had skin problems before when deadlines loomed. I educated her about the likelihood of a skin-stress connection. I also mentioned that her condition might have a specific biological basis that warranted further investigation.

Denise admitted that she had been uncomfortable with her nervousness and knew that her high-strung personality was interfering with other aspects of her life. She decided to begin making changes that would relieve some of her work pressures. For too long she had forfeited things like exercising and other relaxing activities for her job's sake. Denise decided it was time for her to make the first step toward a positive change in her lifestyle which would in turn change her skin as well.

Like Denise, many people must travel extensively because of work. This includes airline attendants, salespeople and executives who live out of a suitcase, miss family members and work on the road. Flying on commercial airlines can be particularly stressful on the skin. In fact, traveling is a situation where emotional stress and environmental conditions combine to produce harsh effects on the skin. Several factors contribute to this problem. A former inspector general of the U.S. Department of Transportation, Mary Schiavo, described some of the deleterious conditions in the cabins of airplanes: poor ventilation which can cause dry skin; unsanitary blankets, towels and tray tables; high-fat high-sodium foods and cramped quarters which make us look and feel poorly.

Here are some healthy travel tips:

- Drink cool bottled water without ice. Do this even when you are not feeling thirsty. Try to drink six ounces per hour.
- Carry a small damp washcloth in a plastic bag. (Washcloths for newborns are great because they are small, soft and thin.) Place over your face and eyes. Afterward, apply a simple moisturizer such as MOISTUREL to your face and hands.
- Bring your own pillowcase and use it.

- Keep your hands off newspapers and magazines. If that is not possible, wash your hands after you finish reading. Try to avoid reading bad news or, alternately, bring a wholesome, enjoyable book or a book of meditations or prayers.
- *Relax.*
- When you arrive at your destination, do not use the hotel soap, which is usually very harsh, but instead carry liquid CETAPHIL or DOVE for your use. Continue drinking water and keep your hotel room as cool as possible.

Skin can *become* stressed from the constant demands of travel. It looks pale, sallow and dry and may have scattered blemishes. It is a condition I have observed on people whose dedication to career and family too often causes them to forget about themselves.

Tess

She came to my office around 11:00 A.M. after arriving on a turbulent red-eye from Los Angeles. Tess had just auditioned for a role in a major film and was rushing back to the East Coast to see her daughter.

Tess is the eldest sister in a family of respected actors, and her success has been the product of hard work and raw talent. Early roles established her as an actress with great range—comedies, romance, adventure, independent films and, more recently, dark dramas. In every part, however, a charming, offbeat personality shines. My impression of her from what I had seen on screen had always been that of a lively, free-spirited woman; however, the person who arrived at my office was anything but. Her skin was dry and ashy. Blemishes covered her forehead and cheeks. She looked exhausted and dehydrated. She told me that she had not eaten all day and that she missed her young daughter desperately when she was away. The first thing I did for Tess was order a large fruit salad and a bottle of water from the deli for delivery to the office.

This had been her fourth coast-to-coast trip in a month. Traveling and stress were making Tess's skin dry and irritated.

Her blemishes were the result of stress overload—too little sleep and a hectic schedule.

I started by treating some of her blemishes. Afterward, I applied a glycolic acid peel to refresh her skin. I have absolute faith in these dermatological methods, but I also know that Tess was benefiting as much from the additional treatment I was providing: a little relaxation, food and water. It seems so simple, and yet quite often we forget to do the bare essentials. We talked while I worked, and her skin seemed to improve as she allowed herself a few minutes to eat, drink and then relax.

We frequently neglect fundamental care in pursuit of what we label more important. We convince ourselves that our tasks can't wait. In the end, our emotions suffer and at some point the stress shows. In some ways we should be grateful when our skin "speaks up." When it does, we can respond accordingly. It's certainly better to suffer with a rash today than have a heart attack or a nervous breakdown tomorrow. We need to treat the immediate skin problems, of course, but more important, we need to respond to our underlying needs.

On the other hand, when good things happen, we should be happy. That's what people say, anyway. The truth is, changes, even positive ones, can cause stress. A great new job, a new baby, a beautiful house, a wonderful romantic relationship can send our spirits soaring. All of these uplifting experiences, however, may leave us a bit frazzled. Perhaps you are lucky enough to positively "glow" when you hear good news, but people with Stress-Reactive Skin might start to feel their skin acting up as they enter a new and exciting phase of life.

Catherine

Catherine, the nervous bride-to-be with several large blemishes on her cheeks, wrung her hands as she explained the necessity of having a perfect complexion by her wedding day. She was one of many women I had seen whose skin had gone a bit haywire right before married life began. It's such a common condition that I call it "wedding skin." Eruptions of adult-onset acne are usually the result of stress and constant touching of the face. Catherine and I established a treatment plan to meet her goals, which would help her feel in control not just of her skin but of the mysterious and wonderful change about to take place in her life. Three weeks before the wedding, she began using a mild antibiotic lotion and started to become vigilant about not touching her face.

The night before her wedding, one stubborn pimple remained, and Catherine paged me. I was at home, but I told her to come to my office right away to meet me. I injected the blemish with an anti-inflammatory solution to shrink the swelling and reduce redness, then I applied a topical antibiotic lotion.

I didn't hear from Catherine until after her honeymoon when she brought in her wedding photos.

"No retouching by the photographer," she said with a smile. "I was so nervous getting ready for the wedding, and it all went so well."

HIVES

You may have heard such expressions as "I got so nervous, I broke out in hives" or "She got hives every time she saw her ex-boss." The common wisdom contained in these phrases indicates that hives and emotions are somehow linked.

Called urticaria in medical parlance, hives appear as itchy red welts with whitish centers. Seventy percent of the cases have no known cause. In general, however, the likely culprits are food, medications and infections. Even water on the skin or blood transfusions have been implicated. Often the welts are migratory, meaning that they can disappear from one part of the body and appear in another. Recurrent episodes of hives which last more than twelve weeks are more common in women than in men. Twenty percent of people with hives continue to experience episodes throughout their lives.

You can expect hives to last for at least two days. Any bout of hives that lasts for more than six or eight weeks is considered chronic.

Treatment. Since the cause of hives is elusive, the treatment is difficult and is aimed primarily at reducing symptoms. Luckily, hives have a short life span and usually disappear spontaneously. This is an excellent example of the body healing itself without any medical intervention.

The following may provide relief: BENADRYL or similar over-the-counter antihistamines. Newer prescription antihistamines such as ZYRTEC, ALLEGRA and CLARITIN can alleviate hives without side effects such as drowsiness. Most creams and lotions are not effective treatments, but cool compresses or SARNA LOTION, available over the counter, provide temporary relief of symptoms.

Cooling down. It is important not to ingest either aspirin or alcohol when you have hives. Standard therapy also calls for the avoidance of excess heat and exertion. I like to take this treatment recommendation one step further. If you have hives, try slowing down and cooling off mentally. By this I mean, take it easy on yourself. Even if you are certain that your hives were caused by something other than stress, you may benefit from making an effort to quiet your mind for fifteen minutes each day. It is well known that decreasing your cutaneous blood flow can reduce itchiness. Relaxing and other stress-reducing techniques such as yoga, meditation and visualization can reduce blood flow when done correctly. What do you have to lose?

Be mindful of your eating habits. Eat several portions of fresh uncooked fruit and vegetables. (Be sure, however, that you are not allergic to any foods before eating them.) Drink cool water and herbal iced teas such as hibiscus or raspberry leaf.

Use visualization and imagery techniques. Visualize your body being cleansed and your skin cooling down. Imagine yourself under a cool, clear waterfall, your skin feeling fresh and rejuvenated. Or visualize that you are floating down a river on an inner tube or sitting at the edge of the ocean with the waves splashing on your feet. As you think of these scenarios, try to pick out details of the scene. What color is the sky? Are there trees nearby that provide comfortable shade? How are you dressed? Are you alone or with someone you love? If possible, have a friend or spouse help you visualize by providing a description of your favorite places. Ask him or her to tell you a wonderful story and let that person take you there in your mind. At first it may seem a bit silly, but you will find that this can be a very pleasant experience.

Imagery or visualization for skin conditions works well if we imagine our skin changing color—from angry red back to its normal healthy tone.

Make an outbreak of hives an opportunity to participate in your own well-being by attempting to relax and treat your skin with care. Having hives is stressful in itself. These relaxation techniques might be just what you need to weather your "skin storm" until it clears.

One or two random cases of short-lived hives have little significance on the emotional level. In cases of chronic urticaria, however, the stress link becomes more obvious. According to psychologists, genetic and environmental factors, along with other emotional variables such as anxiety, depression and personal conflicts, can result in chronic urticaria.

If you suffer from frequent bouts of urticaria, consider whether a stress-related problem may be setting you up for this condition or if other triggers are the culprit.

ITCHINESS

Itching, according to one well-known expert, is the most distressing symptom of skin disease. Generic chronic itching can be created or worsened by stress. In fact, stress lowers your threshold for itching. In other words, the more nervous you become, the more likely you are to feel itchy.

Complex chemical and hormonal processes begin when we are exposed to a stressful situation. These changes can actually make our skin itch. How does your body feel when you react to stress? Do you perspire? Do you feel warm? Can you feel your heart pumping faster? Do you begin to rub or scratch your body? Any of these physical events can cause or worsen itching.

The most common cause for psychologically induced itching is depression. This can occur even when a person claims he or she doesn't feel depressed. Itching can also accompany anxiety.

Here are some clues from *Psychocutaneous Disorders* by Caroline Koblenzer that your itching problem may be stress related:

- Sudden attacks of itchiness rather than a constant level of discomfort

- It occurs after an emotional crisis
- It is worse upon going to bed but seldom prevents sleep
- It is relieved when your attention is diverted

If you suspect that you have a "psychological itch," try some of the stress-reducing activities described throughout this chapter. If this does not help reduce the itching, see your dermatologist.

Skin Tip

The scalp is one of the prime locations for a psychologically induced itch.

Treatment. It may seem impossible not to scratch, but try. Remind yourself that scratching won't make the itch stop, it will make it worse. If you are very itchy and want to avoid scratching, try any or all of these tips:

- Place a cool washcloth or an ice cube over the itchy area and apply gentle pressure.
- Clench your fist gently for thirty seconds, counting slowly.
- Gently pinch or press your fingernail against the itchy area that you otherwise would have scratched.

Even emotionally induced itchiness can be made worse by things in your environment. Try to determine if any of these factors, provided by Jeffrey Bernhard in *Itch*, are contributing to your need to scratch:

- Excessively dry skin; remember to moisturize and not overwash, and avoid hot showers
- Irritating fabrics, especially wool, sometimes polyester
- Contact with formaldehyde resins in permanent press clothing or bedsheets
- Drinking alcohol
- Hot foods

- Using too many blankets
- Alcohol rubs, which may seem to provide relief but only worsen the itchiness
- Static-cling laundry products
- Contact with certain plants such as cactus spicules
- Fiberglas
- Overheating the house; this can cause even people with normal skin to become itchy. The skin loses moisture when the humidity drops below 40 percent. Lower your heater, open a window, use a humidifier or place open basins of evaporating water around the house.

Since itchiness can be worsened by psychological events, it is natural to assume that it can be alleviated to some degree by our mind. One study showed just that. Patients who complained about itchy skin were given a placebo, an ineffective sugar pill. In the study, two-thirds of the patients given the placebo reported some relief from taking the pill. This is not to say that itchiness is all in your mind, but it shows how important the mind can be as a tool to reduce even physically induced itchiness.

PSORIASIS

Psoriasis is a relatively common skin disorder that affects about 6 million people in the United States. Elbows, knees and scalp are common areas for psoriasis, but it can appear on other parts of the body. The nails can even be affected with an appearance of "pitting." Psoriasis is characterized by red skin with overlying silvery scaling. The scales are caused by an overproliferation of skin cells. Its cause is unknown. Psoriasis is usually a chronic problem, coming and going throughout a person's life. Heredity plays a role but is by no means the only factor.

Psoriasis is an inflammatory process, and like other inflammatory diseases, there is the potential for stress to trigger or worsen it. The very latest research confirms suspicions about a connection between stress and psoriasis. Psoriasis is not necessarily *caused* by stress, but there is little doubt that emotional upheavals can worsen it. Continuous stress appears to reduce the response to medical treatments.

In a recent study, patients with psoriasis who listened to meditation tapes during the delivery of PUVA light treatment (a standard treatment for severe psoriasis which combines ingestion of a drug called Psoralen and exposure to Ultraviolet A radiation) were almost four times more likely to achieve clear skin compared with those who received PUVA treatment alone. The meditation tapes instructed patients to become more aware of their breathing and body sensations, and encouraged them to visualize the light slowing down the growth and division of their cells.

Khalid

On a snowy January afternoon, Khalid, a tall man with dark eyes and thick black hair, sat in my treatment room, his feet tapping nervously against the white tile floor. He was referred to me by an internist and had trudged through the snow from that doctor's office to mine. I noticed he was wearing rather lightweight shoes that had become soaked through to his socks.

This is an important visit for this man, I remembered thinking. Even though he had been out in the 20 degree temperature, I noticed that his palm was sweaty when we shook hands.

He told me he had emigrated from Pakistan a year earlier and was just about making a living driving a taxi.

"What can I help you with?" I asked.

With some hesitation Khalid told me that he had had a sore on his penis for the last two years.

"I am afraid that it is cancer. I am afraid that it is contagious, something I can give to my wife. I have been faithful. What could have happened?" The concern on his face asked a hundred more questions.

While I performed an examination, Khalid was silent and still. In a moment I made the diagnosis—psoriasis—a benign, noncommunicable condition. When I told Khalid, he sighed with relief, but it was clear that he was still anxious and overwhelmed.

"I have not had sex with my wife in eight months," he said. "I was afraid I would infect her."

I assured him that sexual relations would not harm his

wife in any way. I prescribed a topical cream that cleared up the problem within a week. My words of reassurance seemed to help as much as the medicine.

Having psoriasis itself is unnerving. Not knowing what it is can be alarming, especially when it shows up in a vulnerable region like the genitals. An emotional state such as Khalid's—anxious, nervous, depressed—can occur among people with psoriasis, although I have seen many who have no psychological distress at all.

The red scaly patches of psoriasis create stress and embarrassment for its sufferers. If the psoriasis is visible, people feel self-conscious. A recent study found that one out of five psoriasis sufferers avoided places or activities because of their skin condition. Three out of four believed that their condition had a negative effect on their self-confidence, and more than half who were polled said they would rather have a more serious medical condition such as hypertension, asthma or diabetes than psoriasis.

The need for chronic care along with an impaired physical appearance undoubtedly has an impact on a person's psyche. The anticipation of rejection by others burdens those with this condition. Worry exacerbates psoriasis, which leads to more worry, and the cycle continues.

Treatment. Typical treatments include steroid creams and ointments, vitamin D creams and lotions (DOVONEX), tar-based products and, more recently, ultraviolet B light plus psoralens (PUVA), SORIATANE and methotrexate.

Emollients, moisturizing baths and antihistamines can often relieve the itching, which can be quite severe. I encountered a patient at the dermatology clinic at New York Presbyterian Hospital who told me his itch was so severe that he had once escaped from jail to get treatment. While it wasn't up to me to decide the veracity of his motives, I can attest to the misery that many people with severe psoriasis endure.

Many people with psoriasis say the best treatment has been a good dose of sunlight and warm humid weather.

Herbal remedies include rubbing mashed avocado on the affected area, licorice extract applied with a soft cloth, drinking milk thistle tea or using a cream containing chamomile that has anti-inflammatory properties.

On an emotional level, I recommend techniques similar to those suggested for the control of hives: Slow down as much as possible. Take time to do nothing at all. Become aware of emotional triggers that might be adding to an outbreak. In addition, support groups, therapy, physician empathy and relaxation techniques can help keep chronic stress-exacerbated psoriasis under control.

ECZEMA (ATOPIC DERMATITIS)

An itchy skin condition that often occurs on the bend of the elbow, backs of knees, wrists, eyelids and lobes of the ears, eczema appears in the form of dry, gray scales and thickened skin with a red background. The medical term for eczema is "atopic dermatitis," meaning an irritation of the skin for which there is no definitively known trigger. People with asthma and hay fever often have a topic dermatitis.

A number of causes can exacerbate eczema. Trauma to the skin and emotional upsets are among the more common ones, but external irritants such as harsh detergents and certain fabrics may also be to blame. Because of its many causes, eczema is likely to occur both in Stress-Reactive Skin and Environmentally Sensitive Skin, which will be discussed in further detail in the next chapter. Atopic dermatitis still baffles us. For years doctors have been trying to identify a relationship between food and eczema, but so far there has been little success.

Some experts believe that "modernization" has led to the rising incidence of atopic dermatitis. This theory is supported by the fact that it is more prevalent in developed countries. Other specialists say that it is more directly related to an imbalance in the immune system.

Few skin conditions have a closer link with one's state of mind than eczema. As far back as the late 1800s scientists have recognized that stress can often precipitate or aggravate an outbreak.

No single test can definitively diagnose eczema. Dermatologists generally obtain information from a patient to make the diagnosis.

If you find that you have eczema and aren't getting much relief from standard therapy, you should consider how your emotions and this condition are interacting. Standard treatment includes topical steroids, moisturizers and the judicious use of topical and systemic antibiotics. Limiting exposure to water and harsh soap is also recommended.

A Word of Caution

If you are annoyed by a skin condition that you think may be caused by stress, you should first consult a dermatologist before making your own diagnosis. Oftentimes, health professionals as well as laypersons chalk up a chronic skin problem to "nerves" and leave it at that. In common medical parlance, stress is called a "wastebasket diagnosis." Even if you are under stress or are a high-strung person in general, you can be suffering from a non–stress-related medical condition that should be treated. Your skin condition may also signal that other health problems are present. Before assuming that your condition is caused by your nerves, consult a dermatologist. If you are still not satisfied, get a second opinion.

TREATMENT

For itching due to Stress-Reactive Skin, especially psoriasis or eczema, several products can provide relief and help you look and feel better.

- A short soak in a cool or tepid AVEENO OILATED BATH soothes skin and spirits. Add three or four drops of lavender oil, known for its calming effects, to the bathwater. NEUTROGENA BODY OIL LIGHT SESAME FORMULA provides a relaxing, wonderful-smelling treat while it moisturizes. You can use it in the bath or shower or apply to damp skin afterward. Beware of a slippery tub.

- To wash your face, use a liquid soap-free cleanser, such as BASIS PURE & SIMPLE FACIAL CLEANSER, FORMULA 405 FACIAL AND BODY CLEANSING LOTION or CLINIQUE RINSE-OFF FOAMING CLEANSER.

- To moisturize, apply EUCERIN LOTION, CETAPHIL CREAM or VASELINE INTENSIVE CARE DUAL ACTION CREAM to damp skin.

- A new product targeted for stressed skin, CLINIQUE SOOTHING CREAM FOR UPSET SKIN, contains hydrocortisone and also comes in a lotion

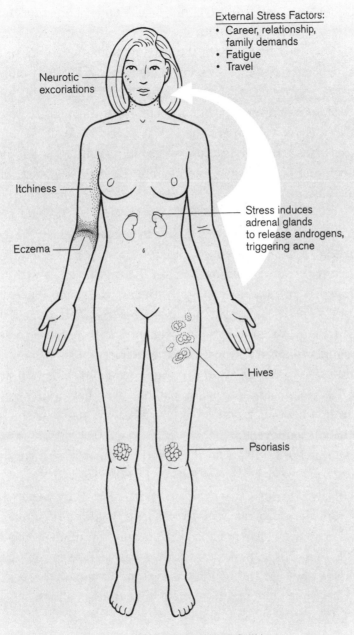

External Stress Factors:
- Career, relationship, family demands
- Fatigue
- Travel

Neurotic excoriations

Itchiness

Eczema

Stress induces adrenal glands to release androgens, triggering acne

Hives

Psoriasis

STRESS-REACTIVE SKIN

A number of skin conditions can be exacerbated by stress. Incorporating stress-reducing techniques can decrease the severity of these skin problems.

for oilier skin. It has a light scent and is oil-free, paraben-free and dye-free. Although you can use it on your face, I find it better for itchy feet, ankles and legs, especially after a shower.

● If you don't have any of the products mentioned above and are anxious for some relief, try this homemade remedy: Mix four tablespoons of instant or regular oatmeal in a bowl with one teaspoon of dried mint leaves. Add hot water and stir into a paste. After the mixture has cooled, apply it to a small area where the itch is present. Cover with a plastic wrap after placing the mixture on your skin. If you feel relief, use it on the rest of your skin for five minutes and then rinse gently with cool water and pat dry.

● KISS MY FACE OIL-FREE ALPHA ALOE provides 5 percent alpha hydroxy and a mixture of plant extracts such as chamomile, yarrow and orange blossom. It is well priced.

● Don't use any eyelid moisturizer. Saturate a cloth with the mixture of one part milk (skim or whole) with one part water. Place the cloth over your eyes and soak for two minutes. This treatment will soothe your eyes and reduce irritation. It is an excellent way to prepare the area for moisturizing. Use a tiny bit of VASELINE or AQUAPHOR and then gently remove the excess with a soft cloth. The eyelids are common areas for eczema. I have encountered many patients who have puffy, red, itchy eyelids from using eye creams. If you have eczema, use only the simplest ingredients on your eyelids.

● During the day, you need to protect yourself from sun damage. Try a two-in-one product such as EXUVIANCE FUNDAMENTAL PROTECTIVE DAY FLUID (for oily skin) or CREAM (for dry skin) SPF 15 by Neostrata. This product contains gluconolactone (a less irritating form of alpha hydroxy acid) and is noncomedogenic and nonacnegenic. You might also try OMBRELLE SPF 15 or ELIZABETH ARDEN'S SUNWEAR DAILY FACE PROTECTOR.

● Use sleepwear and bed linens that are either 100 percent cotton or silk. Allow yourself to luxuriate in their soothing qualities.

● Try not to rush through your skin care routine.

SUDDEN HAIR LOSS
(TELOGEN EFFLUVIUM)

Loss, separation and other personal crises are implicated in a type of sudden hair loss called telogen effluvium. The normal cycle of hair growth is disrupted, and as a result there is a diffuse thinning of hair all over the head. There may also be a stoppage of nail growth as well. Usually, hair loss will follow the stressful event by about one to four months. Physical stress such as blood loss, shock, high fevers, childbirth, surgery and crash dieting can also cause telogen effluvium. There is no real treatment except the gentle handling of the hair. You should also handle yourself with gentleness. Take reassurance in the fact that your hair will definitely regrow.

■ Taking Control of Stress

So far I have been talking about emotions that cause your skin to worsen. Stress provokes some people to touch and squeeze their skin, frequently without realizing what they are doing. This reaction can run the gamut from an occasional urge to pop a pimple to serious mutilation that results in scarring and injury. It is important to recognize these habits as stress reactions and get them under control. In some instances a specific traumatic experience begins the cycle. One extreme case of a stress-induced condition that I recently encountered illustrates this link.

Rosa

Rosa was referred to me by her internist. She was neatly dressed and groomed, but there was little she could do to hide the look of depression in her dark eyes. She told me that she had worked as a waitress at a famous restaurant in upstate New York for many years. Upon examination I noticed a row of deep red sores across her cheek. I knew what they were but decided to talk to Rosa before saying anything about the diagnosis. It took some gentle coaxing for her to unburden herself and tell a harrowing tale.

One afternoon while she was in the ladies' room at the restaurant, an intruder attacked her. He robbed and assaulted her. Rosa fought back and avoided severe harm, but the episode traumatized her. Were the marks on her face the result of the intruder's attack almost a year earlier? Not likely. In fact, Rosa had created the wounds herself, touching and injuring her face over and over in a nervous reaction to the memory of this horrible incident. This condition is called a "neurotic excoriation." In many cases the problem begins when a pimple or rash erupts. The lesion would probably go away on its own, but people with emotional stress react by touching, scratching and digging at their face, many times without realizing what they are doing.

Even though Rosa had caused these wounds, she was desperate for them to go away. She needed healing, emotionally and physically. She wanted to look better and feel better. It took more than a year to clear Rosa's skin. During that time I encouraged her to place an ice cube on her face instead of scratching. If the urge became overwhelming, I told her to call me so we could talk.

Rosa did not want to go to a psychiatrist. I referred her to an internist with experience in posttraumatic disorders who helped her by teaching her behavior modification techniques.

Eventually, Rosa allowed her wounds to heal and began to feel better about herself. The journey to beauty for her was one that began inside and then showed on the outside.

Everyone can use a bit of stress reduction. How to achieve it is an entirely different question. Whatever technique you choose, make sure that it is something you enjoy.

Will it make you more beautiful? It very well might. Feeling composed and in control always enhances the way we look.

My own skin has been affected by stress. In fact, during a busy stressful season, I noticed my skin breaking out. With my wife's encouragement, I began to practice yoga.

If yoga isn't your thing, try stretching for fifteen minutes each morning or evening. Stretching, done correctly, increases flexibility and balance. Stretching also relieves tension and allows you to participate in more strenuous activities with greater ease.

Don't want to do yoga or stretch? How about breathing?

I'm already breathing, you might be thinking. To that I say, "You're not really breathing until you start thinking about it."

A well-known breathing technique derived from yoga provides an excellent pathway to relieve stress.

1   Sit quietly and relax your shoulders. Relax your jaw, your arms, legs, feet.

2   Breathe deeply through your nose, allowing your belly to puff out as it fills with oxygen. Imagine that it is a bellows filling up with air. Breathe down to the bottom of your rib cage, filling your lungs with oxygen. Imagine the oxygen going into your hips, buttocks, legs and/or any part of your body that is sore or in need of healing. If your major problem is skin related, imagine that the oxygen you are taking in is being sent to every pore in your skin, from your fingers to your toes to your scalp. Allow the breath to wash over you.

3   Count to ten as you inhale.

4   If you find it difficult to breathe through your nose, breathe through your mouth and nose. As you exhale, whisper an "ahhh" or "urr" sound, completely emptying your lungs. Then inhale by whispering the same sound or make up a sound.

5   Breathe out through your nose (and mouth) for a count of ten, pushing your abdomen in as the air is released. Imagine that you are exhaling your stress. This is called the cleansing breath. Again, if you have a stress-related skin problem, imagine that your cleansing breath is taking away the irritants and anxiety that affect your skin.

6   As you become more adept at this technique, you can try to inhale for ten and exhale for a count of twenty.

Like yoga, this breathing technique is best taught and demonstrated rather than explained. Take a few lessons from a qualified teacher at a health club, local community center or the Y.

Dr. Richard Fried, a dermatologist and psychologist at Thomas Jefferson University in Philadelphia, considers deep-breathing techniques an important part of treating skin diseases. He believes that of those people who have skin conditions, 50 percent worsen with stress. In addition to traditional medicine and stress-reducing techniques, he advises patients to learn breathing relaxation techniques. His patients have reported significant improvement in conditions ranging from psoriasis to rosacea.

Deep breathing works. You will feel the effects as you improve your technique.

Yoga, breathing and stretching exercises can eventually prepare you to engage in meditation. Meditation is not just for gurus. It is a well-established technique practiced in major medical centers and is recommended for pain relief, stress relief and overall relaxation.

Think about how much you think! All day long, thoughts go buzzing in and out of your head—good thoughts, bad ones, silly ones, sexy ones. You make lists, worry, plan your day, wonder about tomorrow. Your mind is like an incessant wave pounding on the shore. Meditation is about emptying your mind, stilling yourself, becoming quiet. It's about changing your mind from the ocean to a clear lake. Meditation is quite a challenge for most people, but it can really help.

Yoga and breathing methods provide the tools to learn meditation. I learned meditation in college and found that it reduced stress and provided me with a centered and relaxed attitude. Like yoga, meditation is best taught by an expert. It requires that you set aside about twenty minutes each day or at least four to five times a week. Listen to audio tapes such as *Meditation: A Guided Practice for Every Day* (Rudra Press) or *Your Present: A Half-Hour of Peace* (Relax . . . Intuit). For any of these activities to work, practice is essential. Like most exercise programs (or almost anything from playing the piano to scoring foul shots) commitment results in progress and success.

If you aren't interested in yoga, stretching or meditation (don't rule them out until you try), you may enjoy another activity.

Think about an activity that provides you with stress relief, but try to avoid choosing things that are merely distracting such as watching television or talking on the phone. The relaxation response is best done as an exercise inward. In *Inner Simplicity,* Elaine St. James explains that "solitude gives you the opportunity to confront your inner self in a way that few other endeavors can. Out of your times of solitude come serenity, peace of mind and unparalleled opportunities to connect with your soul."

Consider the following stress-reducing techniques:

Gardening. I find pulling out weeds to be both invigorating and calming at the same time. If you don't have space for a real garden, buy some plants and work on them.

Jogging. As I run along the sidewalks or up a path, I try to leave the day's problems behind and just let myself enjoy the passing scenery and the joy of my body running free.

Walking. A quiet walk at the beginning or end of the day is a great relaxer.

Keeping a journal. Write about your worries, dreams and hopes. This is especially comforting for people who enjoy writing. Often when we write things down, such as a list of errands, the tasks seem more manageable. You might also want to write a speech or a letter to a friend, spouse or teacher. You might never send it, but you can express inner feelings that need to be sorted out.

Painting or drawing. Take an art course at a community center or local college. Sitting in front of a canvas or sketchbook and creating something from nothing can be very rewarding. You will be surprised how swiftly time moves as you concentrate on a still life or a face that you are interpreting.

Music. Listening to relaxing music is wonderful, but making music can truly soothe frazzled nerves. Take up an old forgotten instrument. Sign up for a few lessons. Seek out other musicians and try to play a few tunes together.

Experts in the field of Stress-Reactive Skin say that the best results occur when people not only try relaxation techniques but also become aware of the connection between their emotions and their skin. Does this sound a bit extreme for skin care? For a person whose skin reflects inner stress, the answer is no. Ample evidence proves that making a conscious effort to cut down on stress heals the body. There is really no downside to stress-reduction efforts. If you feel as if you are not getting a result, persist. You will maximize the effect of any cream, lotion or medical care by taking the challenge to change yourself from within.

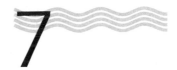

Environmentally Sensitive Skin

- Does your skin tend to break out or develop problems during allergy season or when you use products such as cologne, nail polish and hair spray?
- Is it difficult for you to find skin care products that don't irritate or upset your skin?
- Does your skin react to certain foods that you eat?
- Do insects seem to love your skin, and once you have been bitten, do you find that it is very itchy and painful?

People with Environmentally Sensitive Skin find that their skin changes as a result of contact with many outside elements. While others may have little or no problem with perfumes, soaps and changes in the weather, you, the environmentally sensitive individual, must work diligently to avoid these skin triggers.

Sensitive People, Sensitive Skin

The writer Marcel Proust was a sensitive person, as his writing attests. It seems he also had Environmentally Sensitive Skin. Consider this description by biographer Alain De Botton of Proust's aversion to skin care products:

> *Can't use any soap, or cream, or cologne. He has to wash with finely woven, moistened towels, then pats himself dry with fresh linens. . . . He finds that older clothes are better for him than new ones, and develops deep attachments to old shoes and handkerchiefs.*

Proust had the misfortune of sensitive skin, but the luck of an opulent lifestyle that provided laundresses and handmaids to attend to his needs. A person with limited time and a limited budget need not worry, however. Caring for Environmentally Sensitive Skin can be simple and effective. In this chapter you will learn how you can care for your skin without upsetting it, what products to avoid and what products you can use.

People with Environmentally Sensitive Skin often exhibit other "sensitive traits." For example, you may find that you are affected by other stimuli such as bright lights, noise and extreme temperatures, or even certain unpleasant visual images. You may find it difficult to put something out of your mind once you have seen or heard it. Your sensitivity may make you feel vulnerable. Take the time to understand what upsets you and your skin. Treat yourself with kindness and compassion the way you would any other person.

Your environment is more than the air you breathe. It is food, water, clothing, cleaning products, pollen and dust. It is chemicals found in household items such as draperies and carpets, outdoor pollution, such as car exhaust, and cigarette smoke. These and a host of other culprits can cause any number of reactions or exacerbate preexisting conditions such as acne, eczema and psoriasis.

The number of people with Environmentally Sensitive Skin and the severity of reactions have increased as more pollution, a thinning ozone layer and an abundance of chemicals in our food and water challenge our natural biological defenses. About 1 percent of the general population is allergic to fragrance materials in items such as perfumes, deodorant and aftershave. Men and women are affected equally.

Contact Dermatitis

People with Environmentally Sensitive Skin often suffer from a condition called contact dermatitis. There are two types of contact dermatitis—irritant, the most common type, and allergic.

IRRITANT DERMATITIS

The medical definition of irritant dermatitis is "an inflammatory reaction of the skin caused by an exogenous agent." An exogenous agent is not a spy from a foreign country; it is any outside ingredient, product, chemical or environmental substance that comes in contact with the skin. A wide range of substances and conditions, ranging from plain water to low humidity, can be irritants. A classic example of irritant dermatitis is "dishpan hands." After exposure to hot water, harsh soaps and other chemicals, a person's hands may become red, itchy, peeling or otherwise uncomfortable. This reaction is not an allergy in the true medical sense; your immune system is not reacting to the outside culprit—just your skin. Almost everyone's skin can develop irritant dermatitis if it is subjected to enough irritating agents. Common causes are water, soaps/ detergents, household cleaning agents, fragrances, solvents, acids, oils and mechanical friction.

The best way to treat irritant dermatitis is to identify the triggering substance and avoid contact with it. Many experts believe that steroids are of limited use in treating this condition. You can use a petroleum-based ointment such as VASELINE or AQUAPHOR to soothe the skin. Avoid rubbing or scratching it.

ALLERGIC DERMATITIS

By contrast, allergic dermatitis arises when there is a true allergic response in your body. In other words, after your skin comes in contact with an allergen, your immune system gets revved up and, as a result, your skin reacts. Allergic dermatitis is a hypersensitive reaction in which there is an immune response from within the body. Allergic dermatitis may not be apparent until one or two days or even up to a week after exposure. The classic example of allergic dermatitis is poison ivy. Contrary to popular belief, not everyone has a reaction to poison ivy; only those who are allergic to it develop a problem.

Dermatologists can tell the difference between irritant dermatitis and allergic dermatitis by "patch-testing" the area of the skin that is irritated. Patch-testing involves placing small amounts of potential allergens on the skin and checking to see if there is an allergic reaction on the skin.

Allergic dermatitis accounts for 20 percent of contact dermatitis cases. In general, allergic dermatitis takes place in two phases within your body. In the first phase, your body becomes sensitized to a particular ingredient. When this happens, your body produces "memory T cells" that are primed and ready to respond to a reexposure to the allergen. When reexposed to the allergenic substance, the "elicitation response" occurs, and your skin erupts.

Nickel is a very common cause of allergic dermatitis. About one in seven people is allergic to nickel. People who are allergic to nickel may develop a rash around their wrist, for example, if they wear a bracelet with nickel content. Be aware that nickel can be in zippers, clips, buttons and belt buckles. Other common causes are poison ivy, oak, sumac, rubber gloves, elastic, cushioning, metals in jewelry and tools, topical medications such as neomycin, bacitracin, and benzocaine, semipermanent hair dye, adhesives such as epoxy resins and acrylate, methacrylate monomers, which are used for sculptured nails, and the tolulene sulfonamide formaldehyde resin found in nail polish. Tolulene has been removed from many brands of nail polish, such as REVLON, MAYBELLINE and MAX FACTOR, but not OPI. Check the label. Interestingly, allergy to nail polish mostly affects the eyelids, in and behind the ears, and the neck, due to contact by the nails with these areas. Another common cause is formaldehyde, which is present in some nail hardeners. (Current government regulations require that formaldehyde not exceed a level of 5 percent of free formaldehyde.) There is also the possibility of an allergy to skin products with lanolin. If you suspect that you have a lanolin allergy, use these lanolin-free products: LUBRIDERM DAILY UV LOTION WITH SPF 15 for your face or U-LACTIN HIGH-POTENCY DRY SKIN THERAPY (Allerderm Laboratories, 800-365-6868). Both of these products are lanolin free.

Like irritant dermatitis, the best treatment for allergic dermatitis is uncovering the offending agent and avoiding it. Although this sounds like a fairly simple process, it can be tricky. For example, in more than half of all cases, the diagnosis of an allergy to a cosmetic is suspected neither by the patient nor the doctor. Here is one such example.

Melissa

Melissa came to my office after seeing another dermatologist who had been treating her for a red, flaky rash around her eyes. Although I am not sure what this doctor's diagnosis was, Melissa told me that he had been injecting her troubled skin with a steroid solution. The treatment gave her no relief, and I was concerned about the serious side effects that might result from the overuse of this drug.

I reviewed Melissa's skin care routine and soon realized that she was using a soap and cream that had a high risk for irritation. The solution to her problem was simple: Stop using those products. Within a week her eyes cleared up. As each day passed, her eyes become less puffy and irritated. When she returned to my office, her eyelids were smooth and clear. In her case, the question was not what we could "do" for her but what she could stop doing that would relieve the problem.

I had my own bout with contact dermatitis last year. My hands were red, itchy and peeling. Finding the offending agent was a little like tracking down a criminal. I needed to rule out certain suspects until the "guilty" party was singled out. In my case, it was the latex gloves I used in the office.

Latex allergies are increasingly common among health care workers who are consistently exposed to this product. It may surprise you to discover how ubiquitous latex-based objects are. Balloons, swim goggles, hot water bottles, condoms and underwear elastic contain latex, which may trigger an allergic reaction. A person with a history of childhood eczema, hay fever and/or asthma is also at risk for latex hypersensitivity. Allergies to multiple foods and plants are associated with an allergy to latex. Allergies to avocado and chestnuts have the highest association with latex allergies.

Myths surrounding the causes of and cures for allergic dermatitis may be the reason that many people suffer needlessly. Physicians J. G. Marks and Vincent DeLeo, leaders in the field of contact dermatitis, want patients to know the following:

- Not only costume or inexpensive products cause contact dermatitis. High-priced jewelry and makeup can often be to blame.
- Contact dermatitis does not occur only at the location of the exposure. While the rash may be more severe at the site of exposure, an allergen can be spread to other areas of the body through sweat, touching or scratching.
- A person can develop an allergy to a substance even after using it without any reaction for years.
- Cosmetic allergy is sometimes manifested by mild reactions, such as faint redness and mild scaling of the eyelids.

FRAGRANCE AND COSMETIC ALLERGIES

Fragrances are the most common cause of allergic contact dermatitis from cosmetics. Ironically, perfume and cologne are not the main offenders. Rather, fragrances from skin care products are most often to blame.

Dermatologists and allergists who perform a patch test on patients with suspected fragrance allergies use a "fragrance mix" that contains eight commonly used fragrances. Up to 80 percent of fragrance-allergic patients will have a reaction to this mix.

More recently dermatologists have discovered that fragrances such as ylang-ylang oil, narcissus, sandalwood and jasmine may cause dermatitis, but are sometimes overlooked.

Perhaps you don't even wear perfume or any fragranced product, but you still get occasional rashes on your skin. You should think about whom you last cuddled with. Dermatologists, including myself, have ob-

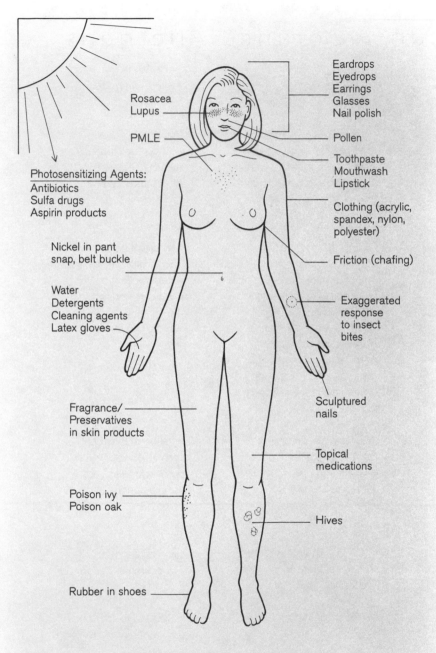

Eardrops
Eyedrops
Earrings
Glasses
Nail polish

Rosacea
Lupus

PMLE

Pollen

Toothpaste
Mouthwash
Lipstick

Photosensitizing Agents:
Antibiotics
Sulfa drugs
Aspirin products

Clothing (acrylic,
spandex, nylon,
polyester)

Nickel in pant
snap, belt buckle

Friction (chafing)

Water
Detergents
Cleaning agents
Latex gloves

Exaggerated
response
to insect
bites

Fragrance/
Preservatives
in skin products

Sculptured
nails

Topical
medications

Poison ivy
Poison oak

Hives

Rubber in shoes

ENVIRONMENTALLY SENSITIVE SKIN

Persons with Environmentally Sensitive Skin may experience allergic and/or irritant
reactions to a variety of substances. They may also find that their skin reacts in an
exaggerated way to sun exposure and/or insect bites.

Common Fragrance Allergens

ALLERGEN	FOUND IN	REACTION
Cinnamic acid	Suntan lotions, balsam peru, cinnamon leaves, coca leaves	Allergic skin reactions, such as hives
Cinnamic alcohol and Cinnamal	Cosmetics such as mouthwash, toothpaste, powder, hair tonics, toilet soap and sanitary napkins. Avoid Crest, Gleem II and AIM toothpaste; colas, sweet vermouth, bitters, chocolate.	Irritation of the skin and perhaps mucous membranes, especially when undiluted
Eugenol	Postage stamp glue; not in cosmetics labeled "hypoallergenic" because of its tendency to cause irritation	May cause gastric irritation and vomiting when ingested; when applied to skin, can cause irritation.
Geraniol	Artificial orange blossom oil, artificial rose oil and many essential oils; also in depilatories to mask odor; omitted from hypoallergenic cosmetics	Allergic skin reactions
Hydroxycitronellol	"Natural" insect repellent products, AVON'S SKIN-SO-SOFT; trademarked under the name Laurine, which is a mixture of water and citronellol	Irritation of the skin; can cause a stuffy nose, hay fever and asthma attacks
Isoeugenol	Perfumes and also in hand creams and in the flavoring vanillin (see also Eugenol above)	Strong irritant; not recommended for use
Oakmoss absolute	Aftershave, perfume	No known toxicity but can cause allergic reactions

(SOURCE: Ruth Winter, M.S. *A Consumer's Dictionary of Cosmetic Ingredients,* 4th ed. New York: Three Rivers Press, 1994.)

served a condition called connubial dermatitis. In other words, you might be allergic to your partner's aftershave or perfume.

Katie

There will always be the diehards who remain loyal to a favorite fragrance no matter what the consequences. My late mother-in-law, Katie, a first-generation Neapolitan, had beautiful olive colored skin, but she was prone to allergic skin reactions. She developed rashes on her wrists and inside her elbows. She suffered with hay fever every spring.

I will always remember Katie generously spraying on Estée Lauder's Youth Dew before going out for the evening. The beautiful pleated bottle with an adorable gold bow was the essence of femininity. Moments later Katie would start to sneeze. Nine times out of ten, an itchy rash crawled up her inner arm. After an especially prolonged sneezing bout, she uttered an Italian expletive that I didn't understand, but I got the point. After the attack, she went on her way. Katie loved that perfume, and nobody could get her to stop using it. After all, it did smell lovely. Sometimes we do have to suffer to feel beautiful.

Other Allergens

Certain types of cosmetic preservatives can cause allergic reactions in sensitive patients. The most frequent preservative sensitizer, Quaternium-15, also known as Dowicil 200, is found in some moisturizers, cosmetics, shampoos, nail polish, mouthwash and fluoride toothpaste. Others that may cause skin reactions are imidazolidinyl urea and diazolidinyl urea, also known as germall II and germall 115; 2-bromo-2-nitropropane-1,3-diol, also known as bronopol. As a matter of fact, bronopol was responsible for so many cases of allergic dermatitis from EUCERIN cream that the manufacturer decided to replace it.

Also avoid, if possible, methyl, propyl, butyl and ethyl parabens and steralkonium chloride.

Most allergic reactions are caused by cosmetics that remain on the skin such as "stay-on" or "leave-in" hair care products or moisturizers, deodorants and perfumes. "Rinse-off" products rarely cause allergic reactions. One exception to this general rule is an ingredient in shampoo called cocamidopropyl betaine. This ingredient is also commonly found in shower and bath gels. In addition, several cases of contact allergy to cocamidopropyl betaine in contact lens fluid have been reported.

Unscented versus Fragrance Free

When looking for products with the least potential to irritate your skin or cause allergic reactions, stick with FRAGRANCE FREE. The word UNSCENTED on a label merely means that the product has no detectable scent, but that may be the result of a masking fragrance. To be extra careful, read the list of ingredients. In some cases, potential allergens such as rose oil and almond oil are put in products and listed as moisturizing agents even though they are fragrances as well.

Treating Allergic Skin Reactions

Treating allergic dermatitis can be a frustrating experience. Doctors use topical steroid creams or oral steroids for severe cases. While steroids alleviate some of the inflammation, unwanted side effects cause some patients to discontinue treatment. In Japan, doctors do not use steroids for this condition because the population has an aversion to the problems these drugs can cause such as acne, unwanted hair growth, thinning skin, as well as more serious medical disorders.

I try to avoid the use of steroids for as long as possible and attempt to educate my patients about avoiding contact with the irritating substance. (See chapter 14 for a discussion of steroids and alternatives.)

AT-HOME CARE

Brief cool showers or baths are best. Use AVEENO bath products if you prefer a bath. Make sure, however, not to stay in the bathtub longer than ten minutes. Never take a hot shower for relief. Doing so will cause your skin to become itchier and raw. Ice cubes placed on the affected skin also work well. Prepare a paste of water and cornstarch, and spread over the affected area. Leave on for fifteen minutes and then rinse with a mixture of two parts milk and one part water. Gently pat dry In addition, BENADRYL or other antihistamine-type drugs can be used if you are very uncomfortable. Beware, though: BENADRYL can cause drowsiness and is best taken right before bedtime.

Photosensitivity

Sometimes the sun and your skin just don't mix well. An excessive reaction to light, most often ultraviolet radiation from the sun, is known as photosensitivity. Many skin disorders such as solar urticaria (hives) are caused by exposure to light. This reaction is known as primary sensitivity. Other conditions can be exacerbated by sunlight. Lupus erythematosus is the most common of these conditions. Photosensitivity can be induced by medications as well. The drug that causes this problem can be a cream or lotion or a pill. An exaggerated sunburn with redness, swelling and blistering are symptoms of a photosensitive reaction.

Natural products can be photosensitizers, particularly lemon, lime, orange or other citrus juice and oils. I know of at least one case in which a woman washed her hair with lemon juice outdoors. A short time afterward she noticed streaks of red irritated skin down her arms and neck. The lemon juice had dripped down her body and reacted with the sun on her skin.

Other photoreactive substances include mangoes, carrots and celery. If you get any juice from these substances on your skin, be sure to rinse off with soap and water before going into the sun. In rare instances people may even get a reaction if they eat abundant quantities of these foods and then go out in the sun.

Ironically, sunscreens can actually cause a photosensitizing reaction. This problem frequently goes undiagnosed because when people get skin reactions to sunscreens, they may believe the product is failing to adequately protect against the sun's rays rather than it is causing an adverse reaction itself. The sunscreen ingredient PABA is a common cause of photosensitive reactions. Other ingredients such as benzophenones, isopropyl dibenzoylmethane and butyl methoxydibenzoylmethane may also cause reactions in persons with Environmentally Sensitive Skin.

HIVES REVISITED

In the chapter on Stress-Reactive Skin, I discussed various stress-related factors that may be responsible for hives. People with Environmentally Sensitive Skin may also have to deal with hives. When hives are induced by sunlight, they are known as "solar urticaria." Within five to ten minutes after being exposed to ultraviolet radiation, itchy welts appear on the skin. Parts of the body that are usually exposed to the sun such as the face and hands may be spared. The condition usually resolves within hours.

POLYMORPHOUS LIGHT ERUPTION

Polymorphous light eruption (PMLE) is characterized by itchy, red bumps and blisters that erupt after sun exposure. Women suffer with this condition more than men. Up to 10 percent of the population in temperate climates, including the United States, have PMLE. People who are exposed to sunlight all year long rarely develop PMLE because they become less sensitive to ultraviolet radiation. Likewise, PMLE appears more often in the spring and fall than the summer. Thirty minutes to a few hours of sun exposure triggers PMLE. Like hives, PMLE usually disappears on its own after a week or so.

Although some people with PMLE are helped with medical treatment, prevention (sun avoidance and the use of broad-spectrum sunscreen) is the best strategy.

LUPUS

This autoimmune disease has many forms, some of which are limited to the skin (discoid lupus) and others which can affect or damage internal organs such as the kidney (systemic lupus erythematosus). It is more common in women than in men. People with lupus are photosensitive. When exposed to sunlight, a "butterfly" eruption may occur over the bridge of the nose and cheeks. Treatment includes conscientious sun avoidance and the use of sunscreen, steroids and antimalarial drugs.

ROSACEA

What looks like acne but isn't? Rosacea. In the early stages of rosacea, you may notice a flushed face that eventually becomes persistently red. As rosacea develops, fine red blood vessels and red bumps or pustules erupt. Unlike acne, there are no blackheads. This chronic condition appears in the central portion of the face and eyelids and is therefore often mistaken for acne.

Rosacea is three times more common in women than in men. People with fair skin are most susceptible, and therefore it has been called "The Curse of the Celts."

While it is unknown what exactly causes rosacea, outbreaks can be triggered by alcohol, spicy food, caffeine, abrasive cleansing, products containing ascorbic acid, extreme temperatures and exposure to sunlight. Some lesser-known food offenders include vanilla, soy sauce and eggplant. I have placed rosacea in the environmentally sensitive section because people with this condition have skin that is "unusually vulnerable to chemical and physical insults."

The National Rosacea Society has recently reported that 82 percent of rosacea patients in a study said their condition was sensitive or somewhat sensitive to common skin care products. Rubbing alcohol was the most irritating topical ingredient. Other ingredients mentioned were witch hazel, menthol, peppermint and eucalyptus oil. Astringents, toners, soaps, exfoliating agents, makeup, perfume, moisturizers and hair spray were listed as the most common irritating products. More than 12 percent of the people in this survey said that shampoo caused flare-ups of rosacea.

Treatment. While there is no real cure for rosacea, it can be controlled. Prescription drugs that keep rosacea in check include METRO-GEL or oral tetracycline. For women who find that rosacea flares during menopausal hot flashes, birth control pills may offer some help.

Eliminating foods that seem to exacerbate your problem and making sure you have adequate sun protection are also recommended. Avoiding alcohol-based cleansers, abrasive cleansers, strong soaps or detergents will definitely help.

Several popular skin care books recommend astringents to treat rosacea. They are wrong. Gentle skin care is essential to keep rosacea in check. If you find that you are still experiencing bouts of rosacea or that it is worsening, see your dermatologist, who will offer effective medications.

Good bets for rosacea are the following:

CLEANSERS
OIL OF OLAY BAR
DOVE BAR

DAYTIME MOISTURIZERS
EUCERIN FOR FACE, SPF 25
OIL OF OLAY DAILY UV DEFENSE SPF 15
PURPOSE MOISTURIZER SPF 15

SUNSCREENS
OMBRELLE SPF 15, waterproof
TI-SCREEN NATURAL SPF 16 (800-PEDINOL)

NIGHTTIME MOISTURIZERS
CANDERMYL CREAM (Galderma)
DML FORTE (Person & Covey)

Daily Sun Protection

Sun protection for Environmentally Sensitive Skin is essential. This includes not only your face but your hands, the back of your neck, and your chest.

No amount of sunscreen will protect you as much as clothing and shade. Too often people have a false sense of security when they wear sunblock. They think they can expose themselves to the sun all day without any harm to their skin. I like to think of sunblock as the equivalent of a condom for safe sex. It must be used properly and all the time, and there is always some risk involved. Absolute sun protection, like abstinence, requires absolute commitment, a difficult task.

For better protection, wear a hat with a three-inch brim and invest in lightweight but closely woven dark long-sleeve shirts, pants and cotton scarves for your neck during the summer. Do your best to stay out of the sun during peak hours of sunlight—from 11 A.M. to 4 P.M. If you plan to be out all day, use an SPF of at least 15, preferably higher. Reapply the sunscreen at least every two hours.

Try these products:
NEUTROGENA SENSITIVE SKIN SUN BLOCK SPF 17
PHYSICIAN'S FORMULA CHEMICAL FREE SUNSCREEN LOTION SPF 25
TI-SCREEN NATURAL CREAM OR LOTION SPF 20 (800-PEDINOL)

Regardless of the SPF in a product, you must reapply it every one to two hours, especially if you are active. Reapply sunscreen immediately after swimming.

General Precautions

LESS IS BETTER

People with Environmentally Sensitive Skin respond best to an austere skin regimen. The fewer fragrances, preservatives and additives in their skin products, the better. Of course, using only the most basic ingredients is not very practical. You don't need to eliminate everything from your skin care regimen. You can still enjoy an elegant and pleasing array of skin care products while keeping irritants and allergens to a minimum. Remember that it isn't only skin care products and certain foods that can cause problems. To avoid other common culprits, I suggest the following:

- Wear cotton instead of wool or synthetics.
- Try to keep dust buildup in your home and workplace to a minimum. Cleaning your floors and furniture with a damp cloth before vacuuming or dry dusting usually creates less dust.
- Rinse your face and hands after you have been in a crowd or have come in contact with potentially irritating substances such as steel wool, pollen or someone else's perfume.
- Change clothing after coming inside from outdoors.

THE DILUTION SOLUTION

The products we use every day are loaded with chemicals, dyes, perfumes and other irritants. Since it is difficult or impractical to entirely avoid contact with everyday items, I suggest an alternative that works for environmentally sensitive people. I call it the "dilution solution."

As the name implies, the dilution solution calls for you to use less or weaker amounts of potentially irritating products. Some suggestions:

- Dilute your shampoo with one part water to one part shampoo.
- To rinse out waxy or greasy buildup from hair conditioners, use a tablespoon of baking soda with half of the amount of your shampoo.
- Use 25 percent less detergent than recommended in your laundry. You can even try cutting down the detergent to 50 percent on clothing that is not stained and add a cup of borax or baking soda to the load.

Recommended products include:
ARM AND HAMMER DYE FREE, FRAGRANCE FREE DETERGENT
ALL-FREE CHEER
LIQUID ULTRA CHEER FREE
WOOLITE HYPOALLERGENIC POWDER
DAWN FREE, a dishwashing detergent that is fragrance free

Cutting down on the amount of detergent you use on your linens can reduce red bumps found on the side of your face that rests against your pillowcase. Scented fabric softeners and detergents are often to blame for this problem. Don't use fabric softeners.

If you simply can't tolerate any detergent, an alternative is a device called the Laundry Disc. It allows water alone to lift dirt and soil. Another product called the Washball can be slipped over faucets or showerheads or put in dishwashers, and will work with water and less detergent for cleaner, healthier results. They can be ordered through Harmony Catalogue (800-869-3446).

The dilution solution will not only help your skin, hair and nails be less irritated but will save you money and preserve valuable natural resources.

A WORD ABOUT NATURAL FABRICS

People with Environmentally Sensitive Skin may find that certain fabrics cause allergic reactions. Dyes and formaldehyde resins are the major source of textile allergies. You can usually tell if your skin reacts to dyes and formaldehyde if you develop a rash on your body that resembles the shape and contour of the garment. To be safe follow these directions:

- Wash new clothing several times before wearing it.
- Avoid tightly fitting garments.
- For people with dye allergies, avoid clothing made from acrylic, spandex, nylon or polyester.
- People who have allergies to resins should avoid all clothing labeled "wrinkle resistant," "chlorine resistant" or "water repellent."

BABYING YOUR SKIN

My daughter, Isabelle, provides a classic example of Environmentally Sensitive Skin. Her skin is lovely but very delicate. She has already broken out with hives after ingesting baby food containing wheat flour. A neck rash flares when she wears any type of collar that is not loose, soft and comfortable. Her eyes were teary and red for hours after my wife applied an unfamiliar sunscreen on her face or when the tiniest bit of shampoo suds dripped into her eyes. If she is bathed too often, her skin becomes dry and prickly. She protests vigorously whenever she is dressed in rayon or anything that is scratchy. A beautiful pair of woolen slippers from Ireland sit unworn on her shelf after she pulled off the shoes and began crying and scratching her feet. We recently discovered that she is allergic to penicillin (like her maternal grandmother, Katie) when she awoke with a hearty case of hives after taking an antibiotic for an ear infection.

With blue eyes, blond hair and porcelain skin, Isabelle needs the simplest products and the most vigilant protection against the elements. If your skin is particularly sensitive, you might want to follow the regimen I use for her.

For bathing (usually every other day): CETAPHIL CLEANSING LOTION. Several drugstores, including Genovese, CVS, Rite Aid and Eckerd, carry their own house brand equivalents of CETAPHIL for less money, and I have found them equally effective.

Moisturizing: JOHNSON & JOHNSON SENSITIVE SKIN LOTION, VASELINE LOTION WITH VITAMIN E and MOISTUREL.

The Not-So-Great Outdoors

SUNBURN

If you happen to get a sunburn, treat it as you would any other burn injury. To reduce discomfort and inflammation:

- Take two aspirins as soon as possible. Continue every four to six hours for a day. Do not go out into the sun again.
- Take a cooling soak. Mix three tablespoons of either cornstarch or baking soda in the bathwater. Stay in the tub no longer than ten minutes. Pat dry your skin very lightly.
- Other home remedies for treating sunburn include mixing equal parts of vitamin A, vitamin E and flaxseed oil from gel capsules, and applying to the skin.

Don't use any soap on your skin. Rinse with cool water only.

After your bath, boil some tea bags, allow them to cool, then apply to any areas that are swollen, such as eyelids. To cool your entire face, apply a mask of plain yogurt; keep on for three to five minutes, then rinse with cool water.

While these remedies will provide some relief, remember that you have already damaged your skin by getting a sunburn. Doing so raises the risk of skin cancers and will contribute to the acceleration of aged skin.

You need immediate medical help if you have a sunburn that blisters and/or have intense pain and/or feel dizzy and/or have very swollen eyes and/or develop a fever. Go immediately to the emergency room or call your doctor.

PRICKLY HEAT

Prickly heat (miliaria) results from blocked sweat ducts and is a common problem for a person with Environmentally Sensitive Skin. Prickly heat usually appears in the form of small red dome-shaped bumps over a part of the body that may have been covered while one's body temperature rose.

Some ways to prevent prickly heat:

- When exercising or working outdoors, wear clothing that "breathes," such as cotton.
- Avoid becoming overheated.
- Drink plenty of cool water to keep your body temperature low.
- If possible, wear a slightly damp scarf or cloth around your neck.

Fortunately, prickly heat usually disappears on its own after a few days away from hot, humid temperatures.

INSECT BITES AND STINGS

After an outdoor barbecue or an early evening hike, are you the one with the most mosquito bites? Do bug bites or beestings result in larger-than-average welts? I have seen a person's ear swell to twice its normal size after a seemingly minor insect bite. These are all clues that you have Environmentally Sensitive Skin.

Patients with Environmentally Sensitive Skin tell me that they find their insect stings and bites to be very irritating. I can attest to the fact that this complaint is not "in their head." It's right on their skin!

Sensitive people should keep their skin covered as much as possible; lightweight clothing is a must when venturing outdoors in the spring and summer. Wear long sleeves and pants if possible. If you are wearing shorts, keep your ankles covered with socks.

DEET (diethyltoluamide) is generally recognized as the most effective active ingredient in insect repellents that protect against mosquitoes and ticks in particular. Many scientific studies report that DEET has a "remarkable safety profile," but I generally don't like to recommend it. I am especially cautious about the use of DEET with small children and pregnant women.

In the United States, DEET is available in concentrations of 5 percent to 100 percent. Experts say that the most effective concentration is 30 percent. Serious side effects in children have been observed following applications in concentrations as low as 20 percent. If you must wear DEET (and in areas where there are significant tick infestations, you might have to), spray your clothing before dressing, not your skin.

Permethrin spray, sold under the names PERMANONE, NIX and DURA-NON, is a somewhat safer chemical-based alternative because it is poorly absorbed through the skin. Permethrin should not be applied directly to the skin or clothing. Use on tent walls or mosquito nets. Skin deactivates permethrin quickly and protection is lost.

Nonchemical insect repellents. Several non-DEET, nonchemical insect repellents appear to be effective at keeping away mosquitoes, blackflies and other bugs, but not ticks. The problem with most of them is that they contain essential oils (most commonly Oil of Citronella) or fragrances that may cause allergic reactions among persons with Environmentally Sensitive Skin. The least allergenic product I have found in this category is BITE BLOCKER (Light Herbal Scent) manufactured by Verdant Brands (800-887-1300). Its main ingredient is soybean oil. One study showed that it provided more than 97 percent protection against mosquitoes three hours or more after application.

Other brands include NATRAPEL, manufactured by Tender Corp. (800-258-4696); AVON'S SKIN-SO-SOFT; MUSTELA INSECT DEFENSE (800-422-2987)—all of which contain citronella, an effective natural insect repellent but one that may cause an allergic reaction in some persons.

Basil leaves rubbed on the body repel bugs naturally. Citrus-scented oils, especially crushed lemon thyme, are also natural bug repellents. In a pinch, light up a few cheap cigars. Many people say bugs can't stand cigar smoke. (I don't blame them!)

Treatment. Once you have a sting or bite, what can you do to alleviate the itching and pain? For itching and irritation, try home remedies first:

- Ice packs and meat tenderizers often do the trick. Mix a paste of unseasoned meat tenderizer and water. Leave it on your skin for half an hour.
- If you don't have meat tenderizer handy, try a paste of baking soda and water.
- Dissolve ALKA-SELTZER TABLETS in a glass of water. Apply with a compress to the skin for twenty minutes.
- Cold apple cider vinegar compresses soothe stings.
- Squeeze the leaves and flowers of a honeysuckle vine and rub into the bites.
- Dab salt on moist skin.
- Herbal remedies include calendula flowers rubbed directly on the skin. Herbalist James A. Duke, Ph.D., in *The Green Pharmacy* suggests making a poultice of garlic and onion and applying it to the skin. You can also take garlic tablets.
- Avoid wearing perfume or floral prints outdoors to reduce the chance of beestings.

Warning

Certain people are highly allergic to bug bites and stings. An anaphylactic reaction, a potentially deadly condition, is most common with bee and wasp stings. If you experience difficulty breathing, have severely swollen lips or tongue, or feel dizzy or nauseated after being stung, go to the emergency room. If you have a history of being highly allergic, ask your doctor about obtaining an "epi" pen. This product contains epinephrine that can be injected directly into the skin and will slow down anaphylaxis.

OTHER SUGGESTIONS FOR STINGS AND BITES

Minor jellyfish stings. Use ice packs and/or take aspirin for pain. Rinse the area with seawater and then soak in vinegar, or baking soda and water.

Fire coral stings. Rinse the affected area with seawater. Use hot seawater compresses or alcohol compresses, and then clean with soap and water.

Sea bather's eruption. An itchy eruption that occurs under swimwear after ocean swimming. Clothing traps jellyfish larvae, which sting the skin. This condition usually lasts about two weeks. When swimming in seawater, especially in southeast Florida, wash your body and swimsuit after leaving the water. Remove your swimsuit before washing your body since freshwater may cause a discharge of larvae. To treat the rash, apply an anti-itch cream and take cool baths in AVEENO OATMEAL BATH.

Bee or wasp stings. If there is a stinger in the skin, it must be removed. Tweezers are best. If that doesn't work, try to remove by gently pressing against the outside of the sting area with a credit card. Do not try to squeeze the area since this will result in pushing the venom farther into the skin. Place a cold compress on the sting to relieve pain. A pocket-sized venom extractor can be ordered through Sawyer Products (800-940-4464) or Terra Tech (800-321-1037).

POISON IVY AND OTHER IRRITATING PLANTS

Seventy percent of Americans are allergic to urushiol, the oily resin on the leaves of poison ivy, poison oak and poison sumac. When exposed to this resin, allergic people often develop an itching, burning, blistering rash. Geographically speaking, you will find poison ivy on the East Coast, poison oak in the South and West Coast and poison sumac in the bogs and marshes of the southern coastal states.

Treatment. Most cases are the result of direct contact with the plant, but if the oily resin gets on clothing, garden tools or pets, and you handle them, you put yourself at risk. People with callused hands are at risk for increased absorption of the resin. Once you have been exposed, wash the area immediately with a strong soap such as DIAL or PALMOLIVE to remove the resin. If possible, splash the exposed area with rubbing alcohol to dissolve the oil. *Do this right away.* After ten minutes, washing will remove only about 50 percent of the resin. After one hour, none of the allergen will be removed.

Once you have removed the resin, you can't spread poison ivy by contact with the liquid inside the blisters on the skin. The lesions themselves are not transmissable or infectious as long as the resin has been thoroughly removed.

You are likely to develop the rash within three days after exposure and will suffer with it for one to two weeks. Apply calamine lotion or BURROW'S SOLUTION to the affected area. Don't use calamine lotion for more than a week since it tends to dry out the skin. Soak in a cool bath with baking soda and gently pat dry. You can also apply a paste of baking soda and water to the area. Cold compresses also work well.

BENADRYL antihistamine can relieve the itching, but it may make you drowsy.

See a doctor if you develop a fever, have very large blisters, the rash is near your face or genitals, or your skin hasn't healed in two weeks.

Do not burn poison ivy plants. Resin travels in smoke and can damage the lungs.

Contact with stinging nettle, which grows in moist woods and along roadsides, can result in hives. Another hive-causing plant is the spurge nettle.

Other potentially allergenic plants include ragweed, dandelion, dahlia, chrysanthemum, sunflower, black-eyed Susan and even such vegetables as endive, chicory and globe artichoke.

At-Home Skin Care for Extremely Sensitive Skin

Just how sensitive is your skin? Does it seem as though anything you put near it causes some kind of reaction? Is your skin always itchy and irritated? If so, I would define your skin as extreme.

Finding lotions, creams, shampoos and sunscreens without sensitizers can be daunting and confusing. I have reviewed hundreds of these products and can recommend only a few. Some must be ordered, so I have provided the telephone numbers. If you have trouble locating any of these products, ask your pharmacist if he or she can order the product.

CLEANSERS

NEUTROGENA FRAGRANCE-FREE LIQUID SOAP

BASIS PURE AND SIMPLE EXTRA GENTLE FACIAL CLEANSER

MOISTURIZERS

DML FACIAL MOISTURIZER WITH SPF 15

DML FORTE CREAM (for dry skin)

DML LOTION (for oily skin)

ELTA SWISS SKIN CREAM (800-633-8872)

THERAPLEX CLEAR LOTION AND HYDROLOTION (800-716-4606)

Other Recommended Products

If none of these products seems gentle enough for your skin, try RO-BATHAOL BATH OIL, formulated without mineral oil, FREE & CLEAR SHAMPOO AND CONDITIONER, VANICREAM CLEANSING BAR and VANICREAM SKIN CREAM and LITE LOTION, all manufactured by Pharmaceutical Specialties, Inc. (800-325-8232). These products are free of many common allergens and irritants such as lanolin, irritating preservatives, fragrance and formaldehyde releasers.

Sunscreens

Most sunblocks and sunscreens contain several sensitizers, and many have ingredients that may cause acne. This list is of the mildest formulations available:

PHYSICIANS FORMULA CHEMICAL-FREE SUNSCREEN LOTION SPF 25 (contains the fewest sensitizers)
ELTA BLOCK SUNBLOCK (800-633-8872)
MUSTELA SUNSCREEN LOTION (800-633-8872)

If you would like specific information about cosmetic ingredients, you can order a handy guide called *International Cosmetic Ingredient Dictionary and Handbook,* published by the Cosmetic, Toiletry and Fragrance Association. It is available at most public libraries and at the Office of the Federal Register, 1100 L Street, Washington, D.C. 20408.

Like a rose, Environmentally Sensitive Skin needs careful attention in order for it to bloom radiantly. In my professional experience, Environmentally Sensitive Skin is often the most beautiful by virtue of its delicate nature. Simple, uncomplicated care is your key to lovely skin.

8

Overexposed Skin

- Did you or do you spend a lot of time outdoors engaging in activities such as gardening, sailing and swimming?
- Are you or were you in an outdoor occupation?
- Do you have light-colored skin, blue eyes, red or blond hair, or freckles?

These are the risk factors for Overexposed Skin. Unlike Hormonally Reactive, Stress-Reactive and Environmentally Sensitive Skin, Overexposed Skin is not an inherent trait but one that develops over time. Your skin has become damaged as the result of long-term exposure to the outdoor elements.

You may have grown up during a time when hardly anyone used sunscreen. The general notion in the recent past was that sun exposure was good for you. It made you look and feel healthy. We now know better. Sunscreen and other precautions remain of utmost importance in avoiding skin damage.

People with fair skin have less sun-protective melanin than persons with dark skin. An African-American woman usually looks ten or fifteen years younger than a light-skinned woman of Celtic or Scandinavian heritage, for example, even if both have been exposed to the same amount of UV radiation.

Signs of Overexposed Skin begin at around age thirty-five. You may have noticed that your hands and face are flecked with light brown spots or freckles. Other places may have a stucco-like appearance. Your skin has lost its "bounce." Fine lines and wrinkles appear around your eyes and lips. These imperfections are showing up now but they probably had their genesis many years ago.

In general, people with Overexposed Skin are not bothered by acne, but they may have dilated blood vessels, especially around the nose or cheeks. Overexposed Skin is not particularly sensitive. As a matter of fact, your skin may have a thicker, coarser texture than that of other people your age.

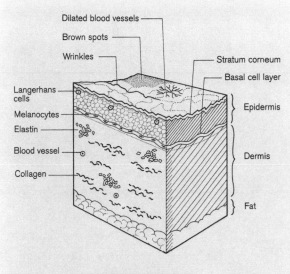

OVEREXPOSED SKIN

In Overexposed Skin there are fewer Langerhans cells, decreased and degenerated collagen, thickened, tangled, degraded elastin, thinner and fewer blood vessels and a diminished fat layer. Coarse wrinkles, sallowness, roughness, discoloration and dilated blood vessels appear on the surface of the skin. The skin is abnormally thin and fragile in some areas and abnormally thick in other areas.

Maureen and Paulette

Maureen and Paulette are sisters, just two years apart in age. They were both born on a small family farm in Pennsylvania. Both have light hair and pale blue eyes. Maureen came to see me when she was thirty-nine. Because of a family history of skin cancer, she needs to be thoroughly examined every year. Paulette, forty-one, also became my patient.

There is certainly a likeness between the two women. As a dermatologist, however, I was struck more by the differences in their appearance. Paulette, the older sister, looks younger than

Maureen by at least five years. Her face is relatively smooth, and she has only the very early signs of aging. By contrast, Maureen's complexion is rough and sprinkled with brown spots. What made all the difference was how these two sisters spent their teenage years and their twenties. Maureen was an avid outdoor person and spent most days helping her parents tend to the farm. At the age of twenty, she married and moved to Bogotá, Colombia, where she began her career as an artist, spending many sunny afternoons painting outdoors.

Paulette shunned the sun. "I was a real homebody," Paulette admits. "I loved reading, cooking, sewing." She also started using sunscreen when she was nineteen whenever she ventured outdoors. Her skin is lovely, and she is often mistaken for the "younger sister."

These two women provide a perfect example of the difference between intrinsically and extrinsically aged skin. They also demonstrate that Overexposed Skin is not exclusive to older people.

Do It Yourself: The Sixty-Day Trial

If you are thinking about visiting a dermatologist or a plastic surgeon to revitalize your Overexposed Skin, wait two months. Why? Because you should give yourself that amount of time to see the difference you can make on your own. Take a "before" picture on day one, then take your "after" picture sixty days later. If you follow some simple daily care as well as the suggestions below, I think you will notice a big difference. If you continue with this care after the sixty days, you will become even more satisfied with the way you look.

Here are the suggestions:

1   *Start wearing sunscreen today and every day.* Do this rain or shine, winter or summer. Get into the habit of applying sunscreen to your face, neck and hands. Depending on what you are wearing, you may also need to apply sunscreen to your chest area and arms.

I encourage my patients to use a moderate amount of sunscreen rather than thick gobs. I think it is unrealistic to expect compliance from patients when they are told to slather themselves in sticky goo every day.

Find a sunscreen that is compatible with your skin. Apply it after you wash your face, while it is still damp. A pea-sized amount is adequate for the face and another two pea-sized amounts, one for each hand. Let the sunscreen soak in.

Stop sunbathing. Don't ever try to get a tan, either in natural sunlight or on a sunbed. It's bad enough that you are exposed to damaging UV rays when you take a walk. If you go to the beach or outdoors for an extended length of time, wear a broad-brimmed hat, UV-protectant sunglasses and as much clothing as possible in addition to your sunscreen. Look for shady areas and spend most of your time there.

If you are outdoors and aren't covered up adequately, use a sunscreen with an SPF of at least 15 or above. Try SHADE SUNBLOCK LOTION SPF 45.

Just because you aren't on the beach doesn't mean you can slack off on skin care. Skiing and hiking have their own sun damage risks. The chance of a sunburn is increased by reflection from the snow. The higher the altitude, the less protection from ultraviolet rays. Wind tends to increase the ill effects of the sun's rays. Wear sunscreen, remembering to also protect your lips with products such as COPPERTONE ALOE AND VITAMIN E LIP BALM SPF 15 or NEOSTRATA AHA LIP CONDITIONER WITH SPF 15.

Stop smoking. If you smoke, stop right now. The damage that smoking can do to your skin was revealed in a recent study of identical twins in which one smoked and the other didn't. Of the twenty-five twin sets, the smoking twin consistently had older-looking skin than the nonsmoking sibling by as much as 40 percent. Tobacco may wreak havoc by constricting blood vessels, damaging the gene repair processes or stimulating the release of enzymes that dissolve the skin's elastic components. Whatever the underlying biological causes, smoking shows up on your face.

Smoking also contributes to skin problems in these ways:

- Slows down wound healing, a big problem if you are considering any kind of plastic surgery.
- May result in wider, bigger scars once the wound has healed.

- Decreases vitamin A absorption, which contributes to wrinkles.
- May have an influence on psoriasis.
- Is a contributing factor in melanoma, the deadliest skin cancer. Smokers are also likely to have melanoma spread to other parts of the body.
- Contributes to lip cancer and gum disease.

Smokers purse their lips and squint when they take a puff. Eventually, these expressions become etched on the face—deep vertical lines on the upper lip and crow's feet around the eyes.

I haven't even discussed the well-known health risks associated with smoking: lung cancer, emphysema and heart disease. But you have the picture. If you are inspired to quit for the sake of your looks alone, you have my blessings and congratulations. There are many ways to stop, but nothing works better than cold turkey. Avoid people who smoke and, if possible, the places where you enjoyed smoking. Contact the American Lung Association and the American Cancer Society for more information about smoking cessation programs.

Sleep tight. Begin to treat your sleep like any other health priority. Convince yourself that you must get between seven and eight hours of sleep every night. Stick to a schedule that doesn't vary by more than half an hour even on the weekends. You have to give your body and your skin an opportunity to replenish itself. You can't do this if you are always "on." Would you run your car nonstop and expect it to be in top shape at the end of the year?

If you have trouble sleeping, consider whether any of these factors are interfering with the rest you and your skin need:

- Too much noise or light in your bedroom.
- Too hot in your bedroom.
- Not getting enough exercise during the day (but be careful not to work out too close to your bedtime).
- Eating heavy meals before bedtime or not eating enough during the day.
- Drinking alcohol. Yes, alcohol can make you sleepy, but it can also interfere with the quality of your sleep. It is also dehydrating, which can affect the way your skin looks.

- Daytime napping.
- Caffeine—a big culprit. Coffee, tea, chocolate, cola drinks, Mountain Dew and some aspirin products contain caffeine. Avoid especially after three in the afternoon.
- Not winding down. It's unwise to jump into bed if you haven't given yourself time to relax. And watching television isn't the best way to do that. Newscasts with reports of horrible crimes and tragedies, tense melodramas and noisy sitcoms don't soothe anyone's nerves. Try listening to some nice music, reading or writing a letter before bedtime. Or how about a nice peaceful conversation with the person you live with or a pleasant brief phone chat with someone you know who needs a little company?

5 *Relax your face.* During the sixty-day trial, begin to become aware of the way you move your face. Do you scowl, frown or make other exaggerated facial expressions? Place a mirror in front of you while you are on the phone and take note of how you use your face while speaking. Pronounced facial expressions put wear and tear on your face. A passage from an 1870 beauty book advises women to "avoid frowning and grimaces which contract the muscles of the face." It is still good advice. Do not sit by a bright light that forces you to squint.

Become mindful of the times when you make faces such as when you are worrying or angry. Place two fingers on the area that's "scrunched" and smooth out the scowl with light strokes across the face. Think of how your face looks when you are restful and relaxed, and try to maintain that look as much as possible.

At-Home Skin Care for Overexposed Skin

Cleansers

Stop using any kind of soap or soap-based products on your face. They are too drying and will accentuate wrinkles. Instead, use cleansers such as CETAPHIL CLEANSER.

You should also be using alpha (or beta) hydroxy or salicylic acid. Wet your face and then gently apply the AHA cleanser. If you experience a slight tingling, don't worry. Just wait thirty seconds and rinse well. Avoid getting any of these products in your eyes or mouth.

NON-AHA CLEANSER/MAKEUP REMOVER

DECLEOR CLEANSING OIL

ALMAY MOISTURIZING GENTLE EYE MAKEUP REMOVER

PRESCRIPTIVES EYE MAKEUP REMOVER, which is less oily

Don't rub your face, especially under your eyes, to remove makeup. Instead, gently apply the makeup remover and let it set for a minute or two. Remove with a soft damp cloth.

And remember: you usually don't need to wash your face in the morning if you washed it before bedtime. Just splash a little water on it and pat dry in the morning. Follow with a moisturizer while your face is still damp.

For your daily shower or bath, try NIVEA SHOWER AND BATH SKIN RE-NEWAL GEL, a nonirritating blend of two AHAs (lactic and citric) along with chamomile extracts. Alpha-hydroxy–based bathing products are especially useful for smoothing arms and legs.

Moisturizers

For a simple routine, try these moisturizing sunscreen products during the day:

PHYSICIANS FORMULA SUN SHIELD SPF 20

AVEDA DAILY LIGHT GUARD SPF 15

LANCÔME SPF 25 SUN BLOCK FACE CREAM

For extra eye protection, use KIEHL'S ULTRA MOISTURIZING EYE STICK WITH SPF 18.

Another effective method is to mix one part non-SPF moisturizer and one part sunscreen in your hand and then apply lightly over the face.

EVENING MOISTURIZERS

If you find that nightly application of an alpha-hydroxy-acid product is too irritating (you probably won't), alternate every other night with a cream such as

ELIZABETH ARDEN EIGHT-HOUR CREAM

VASELINE PETROLEUM JELLY CREAMY FORMULATION

ALPHA HYDROX NIGHT REPLENISHING CREAM (CONTAINS NO AHAS)

If your skin tends to be very dry, a twice-weekly "slathering" of the products mentioned above will leave your skin very soft. Dampen the skin with warm water and pat dry. Apply a generous amount, then cover your face with a slightly dampened towel for a few moments. Tissue off, then rinse lightly with warm water and pat dry. Doing this to your skin provides it with a type of moisturization called "occlusion" which helps skin retain its natural moisture.

THE EXTRAS

The information above is the blueprint for effective care of Overexposed Skin. I have tried to make it as simple as possible while focusing on maximum results. What follows are some extra bits of advice that can do even more to make your skin look younger faster.

Retin-A wanna-bes. Because prescription products like Retin-A have become so well known and well regarded, a lot of companies have created an over-the-counter product that sounds like Retin-A but isn't. Retinoic esters such as retinyl or retinyl linoleate (derivatives of vitamin A) do show promise for smoothing the skin. (See page 244 for specific product recommendations.) If you are interested in faster results, you may want to consult a dermatologist about using Retin-A.

Nutrition. Your entire body benefits from good nutrition, and your skin is no exception. Be aware that alcohol and caffeine are very dehydrating. Your skin will begin to look parched, crepey and gray if you overuse these water-and-nutrient thieves. They also put an extra strain on vital organs such as your liver, kidneys and brain.

Drinking six to eight glasses of water a day cleanses the system and allows it to function with greater ease. To help you keep track of the amount you should be drinking, it's a good idea to premeasure your "water goal" in one large container or several small ones and place them in the refrigerator. Along with adequate water, your body needs fiber to keep your complexion looking its best. Many high-fiber foods are rich in essential vitamins and antioxidants. In addition, fiber works to keep your body hydrated and to flush away toxins.

Treat yourself to a fresh vegetable juice drink at least twice a week. Mix fresh raw celery with carrots, apples and a little ginger—and enjoy. Experiment and find a mix of fruits and vegetables that you like. Add bananas for potassium and fresh tomato for rich skin nutrients. You will feel more energized and may even notice a change for the better in your skin.

If you have done your very best during your sixty-day trial, take another photograph of yourself. Try to use the same lighting, hairstyle and facial expression. You should notice a difference. If you are pleased with the result, maintain the regimen for another thirty days. You will see even more improvement.

If you are still looking for a little bit more, make an appointment with a dermatologist to find out what he or she can do for you. Knowing that you have done your very best gives you a great head start in your path to beauty.

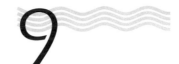

9

Hearty Skin

Lucky you! Your skin looks great, and you probably don't even spend too much time taking care of it. You probably look better than most people your age. You rarely have allergic reactions to skin products and need only the simplest routine to look great. Why are you so fortunate? The most obvious answer is that you won the gene pool lottery. Did your parents and grandparents have smooth, lovely skin? Women with Hearty Skin are often from Mediterranean backgrounds and may have an olive complexion. Many African-American and dark-skinned Hispanic women are blessed with Hearty Skin. Fair skin can sometimes be of the hearty variety, but it usually shows the signs of aging sooner than darker skin.

If your skin is light brown or darker, it can still become sun damaged, albeit at a slower pace than a fair-skinned person's. A sunscreen with an SPF 8 used daily is adequate unless you have a particular sun sensitivity, such as dark splotches, healing acne or any other healing wound on the face. Medical conditions such as lupus may make your skin more vulnerable to sun damage. If that is the case, you should select an SPF of 15 or greater for daily use.

Some Sunscreen Recommendations

ELIZABETH ARDEN SUNWEAR DAILY FACE PROTECTOR
L'ORÉAL PLÉNITUDE ACTIVE DAILY MOISTURE LOTION SPF 15 for daily wear
SHISEIDO TRANSLUCENT SUNBLOCK STICK SPF 30

Cleansers

Use DOVE or CLINIQUE facial soap, or OIL OF OLAY FOAMING FACE WASH. You should clean your face once a day, preferably before bedtime. In the morning, a splash of warm water will be enough.

Moisturizers

Even Hearty Skin needs care to keep it looking beautiful. You can use relatively inexpensive but nourishing moisturizers.

If your skin is on the dry side, try:

ESTÉE LAUDER DAYWEAR
ELIZABETH ARDEN VISIBLE DIFFERENCE
CLINIQUE DRAMATICALLY DIFFERENT MOISTURIZER

If your skin tends to be oily, try:

AVON ANEW ALL-IN-ONE OIL-FREE PERFECTING LOTION
OIL OF OLAY AGE-DEFYING PROTECTIVE RENEWAL LOTION
PRESCRIPTIVES ALL YOU NEED OIL-FREE ACTION MOISTURIZER

For overall body care, you can use practically any moisturizer that doesn't irritate your skin. Just remember to moisturize after every shower. Some good inexpensive choices are VASELINE INTENSIVE CARE MOISTURIZING CREAM, NEUTROGENA BODY OIL SESAME FORMULA and AVON MOISTURE THERAPY BODY LOTION. If you want to splurge a bit, try ESTÉE LAUDER RESILIENCE BODY.

If the skin on your body is rough, ashy or discolored, you should try a moisturizer with an alpha hydroxy acid for the body, such as EUCERIN PLUS ALPHA HYDROXY MOISTURIZING CREAM. I often recommend this product to dark-skinned women who have problems with dry legs and arms, knees, elbows and sides of the feet.

A nightly moisturizing routine will keep your skin looking great. If you are over thirty-five, you may want to consider using a product containing alpha hydroxy acid, at least every night.

AHA Moisturing Night Creams

M.D. FORMULATIONS FACIAL CREAM
POND'S AGE DEFYING COMPLEX

Overlapping Skin Types

Now that you have finished reading about the five Skin Profiles—Hormonally Reactive, Stress Reactive, Environmentally Sensitive, Over-exposed and Hearty—you have probably been able to identify yourself. For some of you, however, the characteristics of more than one Skin Profile may define your skin. As I have stated throughout this book, these Skin Profiles are not meant to lock you into an inflexible skin care routine or define your skin in absolute terms. Instead, my goal has been to provide you with a framework that will help you to determine the essential features of your skin instead of merely reacting to its changes.

If you haven't already done so, I would advise you to read about all of the Skin Profiles. Doing this is important because your skin is likely to change over the years or seasons or through various life events. You may even be able to prevent some of the unwanted characteristics from other Skin Profiles.

Some general guidelines for persons with overlapping skin:

Acne breakouts, whether hormonally or stress induced, have common characteristics and can be treated with many of the same products. The most important issue is determining *when* your skin has a propensity to break out and working with that information to keep pimples from developing.

If your skin fits within the Environmentally Sensitive Profile but you struggle with acne and/or signs of aging, the essential principle that should guide you is the use of gentle, nonirritating products.

3 The most important consideration for every Skin Profile is protection from the sun, gentle handling of the skin and consistent daily care.

4 Experiment. Select what is most compatible based upon my recommendations. Determine what is working for you and what isn't. Introduce your skin to one new product at a time. Try something new for a few days before trying another product.

The most important adjustment you can make to your skin care routine involves your attitude. Scanning the cosmetic counters for a miracle cream that instantly provides results won't work. Instead, your goal should be an increased awareness of how your skin reacts. Become mindful of what is going on inside and outside your body and how that affects your skin. With some effort, you will be able to gain control and you will notice that your skin is looking great and a new and more confident person is emerging.

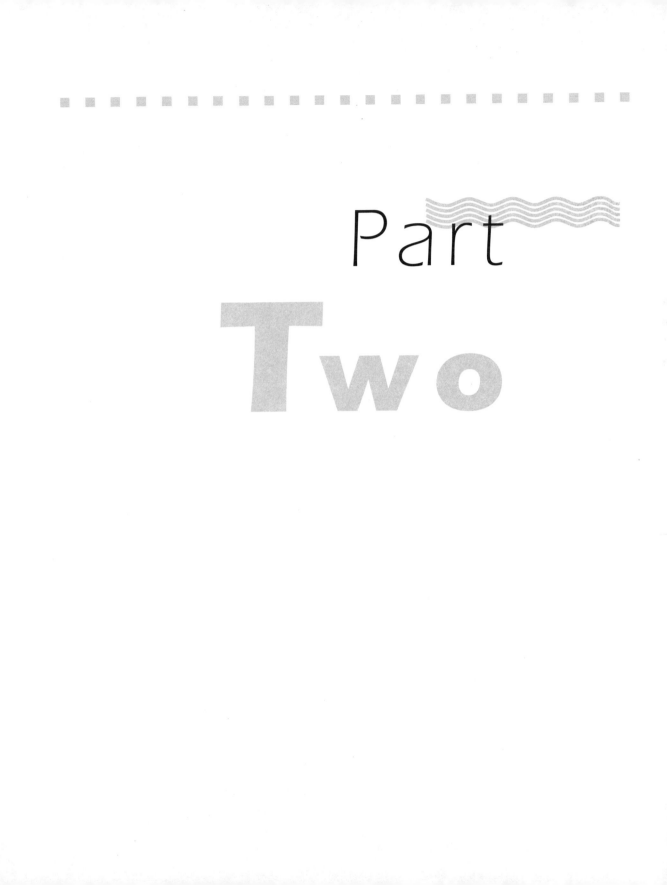

Part

Two

10

"Doctor, what should I buy?" Patients ask me this question every day. They want to know what kind of soaps, moisturizers and cosmetics they should use for good-looking skin. Many of them have medicine chests full of last year's "groundbreaking" skin treatments, only to be lured by a new "breakthrough" that promises even better results. Skin care advertisements make claims that sound like miracles. We want skin that "glows," that is "luminous," that is "visibly younger."

Even the most sophisticated consumer can be tempted by the possibility of recapturing youth. Is anyone making sure the promises are true? Can we rely on the integrity of the cosmetic companies to tell us all we need to know about the products we are so eager to buy?

In this chapter, I will provide you with a brief description of the regulation of cosmetics and how you can become an informed consumer regardless of your Skin Profile.

■ A History of Regulation

Today, the Food and Drug Administration oversees the sales of cosmetics, among other things, and the Federal Trade Commission regulates claims made in their advertisements under the Fair Packaging and Labeling Act. Considering that Americans spend $30 billion annually on cosmetics, there certainly does seem to be a need to control and monitor this business.

In the early part of this century, women literally risked their lives to look beautiful. The first face powders in America were blends of lead and arsenic salts. Eyelash dyes, compounded with aniline dye, blinded and disfigured a woman in 1933. A depilatory cream called Kormelu contained rat poison. One nineteenth-century beauty book recommended this treatment for excessively large breasts:

> *The breast can be readily reduced by constant inunction of an ointment of cadmium or iodine, the administration of iodine internally, and . . . firmly applied bandages of adhesive plaster.*

To combat "dandriff" and other scalp maladies, the same author recommended an ointment containing powdered borax, a dilute solution of lead, clean lard and a few drops of rosewater. For those who wanted whiter teeth, a mixture of powdered brick, cuttlebone and pumice did the trick.

With no governmental body overseeing the distribution of these products, ingredients could be not only ineffective but harmful. With the support of Eleanor Roosevelt, women's groups and consumer activists, the Federal Food, Drug and Cosmetic Act was passed in 1938. Its main thrust was to make cosmetics safe for use through federal regulation.

Historians tell us that cosmetics, creams and powders became an "aesthetic expression woven deeply into women's daily life" by the 1930s. Despite some early bad publicity, "women did not renounce make-up, for it had become the common language of self-expression and self-understanding."

Drug or Cosmetic?

Are cosmetics just lipstick, blush and eye shadow? What about deodorant, vitamin C creams, and alpha hydroxy acid? According to the U.S. Food and Drug Administration, the definition of a cosmetic is any product "intended to be rubbed, sprinkled, sprayed on, introduced into, or otherwise applied to the human body or any part thereof for cleansing, beautifying, promoting attractiveness or altering the appearance." This definition embraces hair dye, shaving cream and talcum powder, for example.

Products deemed cosmetics do not require preclearance for safety or the demonstration of efficacy. This relatively loose regulatory scheme gives companies a wide range in which to describe the wonders of their potions and lotions. Companies cut down on lots of red tape if what they are selling is determined to be a cosmetic. The FDA does require, however, that a cosmetic not be adulterated or misbranded.

By contrast, drugs are defined as "articles intended for use in the diagnosis, cure, migration, treatment or prevention of disease in man or other animals. Articles (other than food) intended to affect the structure or function of the body of man or other animal." Regulators impose a much more rigorous safety and efficacy process for a product once it is determined to be a drug. The approval process can be expensive and time consuming.

Some cosmetic preparations, regulated like drugs, are classified as "over-the-counter drugs" because they are used to both enhance appearance and prevent disease. Toothpaste, dandruff shampoo and sunscreen, for example, fall within this category. An easy way to tell if you are buying an over-the-counter drug is to see if the first ingredient is listed as an "active ingredient."

Whether the product is used for beauty, health or a combination of the two, it must bear a label with a "declaration of ingredients." This list must contain the product's ingredients in their descending order of predominance (actual concentration in the product). Anything that represents more than 1 percent of the product must be listed.

Consumers often get the impression that Europe is far ahead of the United States in developing beauty products. In reality, Europe lags behind when it comes to listing ingredients. Cosmetic ingredient labeling was introduced in the United States twenty years ago. It wasn't until 1997 that the European Cosmetics Directive began requiring that all cosmetic products marketed in Europe display their ingredients on the outer package.

◼ Stepping Over the Line

Government watchdogs can and do crack down when cosmetic companies step over the line. In an effort to ensure the utmost fairness, the courts have held manufacturers to a strict standard: When making claims, they must consider Jane or John Q. Public an "ignorant, unthinking and credulous consumer." While this may sound a bit insulting to you, it's at least a way to keep the cosmetic business honest.

When cosmetic manufacturers try to have it both ways—they want a product to be both a drug (in terms of the claims they can make) and a cosmetic (in terms of how the article gets approved)—the FDA steps in. In many ways the legal distinction between a drug and a cosmetic depends on the claims made rather than the ingredients within it.

When several cosmetic companies stepped over the line in the late 1980s, the FDA said it would not tolerate two-sided claims. In 1986, Dr. Christiaan Barnard, the South African heart surgeon, developed the Glycel skin care line. Ads for the product touted that with the use of Dr. Barnard's Cellular Anti-Aging Cream "normal functions of the cell will return, allowing the skin to look younger." Other cosmetic companies, eager to sell the public their versions of a youth cream, began pushing similar products with similar promises.

The FDA began sending warning notices to dozens of cosmetic company giants, including the makers of Glycel. They told the manufacturers that claims of "increased collagen," "anti-wrinkling," "enhanced cellular function" and other "structural repair" placed their products in a drug category. As such they would be subject to the more stringent scrutiny. The parties reached a settlement, and the companies agreed, among other things, not to claim that their products slowed down or reversed the aging process. Nor could they claim that the products provided permanent results or that they affected the skin below the epidermis.

An earlier example of the drug-versus-cosmetic controversy occurred in the 1940s when manufacturers began claiming that placenta (the tissue surrounding a fetus) provided beneficial effects for the skin, such as stimulating tissue growth. The regulatory agencies pounced on these claims and insisted that a product using placenta should be classified as a drug. Manufacturers changed their tune and dropped their claims. Placenta is still used in cosmetics as a protein source, but with none of the earlier hype.

On the safety front, the FDA and state agencies intercepted a cream from Mexico, Crema de Belleza, in 1996 after an investigation revealed that the product contained 6 percent to 10 percent of mercury by weight. No harmful effects were reported resulting from use of this product.

Despite the FDA's relatively liberal policy, few real problems occur because the industry tends to regulate itself. The manufacturers realize that it isn't smart business to sell a harmful product or one that doesn't provide at least some kind of benefit.

In 1972 a cosmetics trade association requested that the FDA establish the Voluntary Cosmetics Registration Program in which companies could submit information on products, including reports of adverse reactions. With this information the FDA would be able to maintain a database about ingredients in products. About 50 percent of cosmetics companies participated. Budget cuts recently forced the FDA to eliminate the program. The FDA now advises consumers who are experiencing an adverse reaction to a cosmetic to call the Cosmetic Adverse Reaction Monitor at 202-205-4706.

Cosmeceuticals: A Hybrid

The line between cosmetic and drug is blurring. In fact, the word "cosmeceuticals" has evolved to describe products that don't quite fit the definition of either drug or cosmetic. The word "cosmeceutical" is not an official category within any regulatory scheme, however, and it is not recognized by the Food and Drug Administration.

The largest category of so-called cosmeceuticals is alpha hydroxy acids (AHAs).

The FDA's concern about AHAs revolves around the lack of long-term safety testing of these products. Potential problems include skin irritation and increased sensitivity to sunlight, and it is not known whether long-term chronic low-grade irritation will have adverse lasting effects.

The Cosmetic Ingredient Review Board, an independent panel of physicians with no financial ties to the cosmetic industry, investigated the safety of AHA. The board determined that AHAs are safe as over-the-counter products in formulations with less than a 10 percent concentration and a pH of 3.5 or greater. Trained salon professionals could safely apply AHAs with a concentration of 30 percent or less and a pH of no less than 3.0.

These recommendations, while not yet laws, will help ensure that AHAs are used safely and with good results.

Men and women have used alpha hydroxy acid for centuries to clear, cleanse and exfoliate the skin. In the 1700s ladies of the French court dabbed aged wine on their faces to soften their complexion and remove unwanted spots and blotches. Back even further, in 1560 B.C., physicians used plant, animal and sulfur substances for exfoliation. In 1974 the term "alpha hydroxy acid" was introduced for the treatment of a severe dry skin condition called "ichthyosis." Newer technology allows doctors and consumers to use these ancient recipes in a stronger but more predictable formulation to benefit the skin.

AHAs occur naturally in foods: citric (citrus fruits), lactic (sour milk), malic (apples), tartaric (fruit and grape wine) and glycolic (sugarcane). Glycolic acid has a small molecular size and is very adaptable for cosmetic use because of its ability to penetrate the skin. AHAs are a true drug/cosmetic hybrid. They provide some superficial effects, such as hydration, but they also change the structure of the skin in the same way a drug would. AHA products slough away layers of dead skin, cells that build up to form an overly thick stratum corneum.

At least one study has shown that the continued use of products containing a 25 percent concentration of AHAs can increase collagen production. AHAs also increase the number and quantity of elastin fibers and tighten the superficial skin layers.

One of the most frequent questions I hear from patients who are using AHA products is "Do I have to stay out of the sun?" To which I reply, "Don't you already do that?"

Using AHAs makes your skin more sun sensitive, and you must be vigilant about the daily use of sunscreen on your face, winter and summer. Do not sunbathe even if you are using sunscreen. Wear a hat if you plan to be outdoors on a sunny day. If you follow basic skin protection precautions, your skin will not suffer. If for any reason you plan to be out-doors for a lengthy period, discontinue your AHA regimen for two weeks prior to that time.

AHA Tips

1 Stick with lactic or glycolic acids when using AHAs. These two types have undergone the most rigorous testing for both safety and effectiveness.
2 Don't be fooled by similar ingredients such as sodium lactate, sugarcane extract, mixed fruit acids and fruit extracts. They won't exfoliate.
3 Wait ten minutes after cleansing to apply any AHA or salicylic acid. Moisture on the face can dilute the effects of the acid.

EFFECTIVE FORMULATIONS

AHAs are most effective at a low pH, but they can also be irritating to the skin at that level. At a higher pH they are milder and less likely to cause irritation, but they lose effectiveness. According to experts, the most effective pH range is between 3 and 5. A product formulated at a lower pH will contain a higher amount of free acid and will penetrate faster than a similar product having a higher pH.

AHAs and Your Skin Profile

Higher concentrations of alpha hydroxy acid products are needed to treat Overexposed Skin. For people with sensitive skin, the right for-mulation of alpha hydroxy acid can actually make the stratum corneum more resistant to irritation from products such as detergents.

Of the products listed on page 186, the best choices for your Skin Profile are as follows:

For Hormonally Reactive Skin: ALPHA HYDROX EXTRA STRONG OIL-FREE. In general, people with oily and acne-prone skin should use alpha hydroxy acids with a concentration of about 8 percent to 10 percent once in the morning. At night you can repeat the application of the glycolic acid cream. For relief of rough dry skin, I recommend a concentration of 15 percent.

pH of Popular Alpha Hydroxy Products and AHA Concentration Where Available

PRODUCT	PH	AHA %
*Alpha Glow	4.8	8
*Alpha Hydrox Enhanced Lotion	4.0	10
*Alpha Hydrox Extra Strong Oil-Free	3.9	10
*Alpha Hydrox Face Cream (Normal Skin)	3.9	8
*Alpha Hydrox Sensitive Skin	4.1	5
*Camocare Gold-Chamomile Face Lift	3.8	
*Exuviance by Neostrata	3.8	8
Formula 405 AHA Facial Day Cream	2.7	
LactiCare Lotion	5.6	
*L'Oréal Plénitude Excell A3	3.8	
*Neostrata Exuviance Evening Restorative Complex	3.8	8
*Neostrata Exuviance Fundamental Multi-Protective Day Crème and Fluid SPF 15	3.8	4
*Neostrata Exuviance Multi-Defense Day Cream and Fluid, SPF 15	3.8	8
*Neutrogena Healthy Skin Face Lotion	3.3	
*Pond's Age Defying Complex	3.8	
*Pond's Age Defying Lotion for Delicate Skin	3.7	
Purpose Alpha Hydroxy Moisture Cream	5.5	8
*Sally Hansen Skin Recovery	4.3	

*Falls within most effective pH range.

For Stress-Reactive Skin: CAMOCARE GOLD-CHAMOMILE FACE LIFT. The soothing ingredients in this product give stressed-out skin a boost.

For Environmentally Sensitive Skin: ALPHA HYDROX SENSITIVE SKIN or POND'S AGE DEFYING LOTION FOR DELICATE SKIN

For Overexposed Skin: Pond's Age Defying Complex (8%). A good basic product that is perfect for use at home. People with Overexposed Skin should see a dermatologist for stronger AHA treatment.

For Hearty Skin: Alpha Hydrox Face Cream (Normal Skin). Inexpensive and unlikely to create any problems. Will smooth out early wrinkling and improve texture.

Does It Really Work?

It's human nature, I suppose, to want something exotic, different, out of the ordinary. Because of this, manufacturers of creams and lotions hold us in a perpetual spell when they tout new ingredients that sound either scientific, natural or both. I think it's critical for you to understand what you are paying for. You will then begin to realize that the basic stuff does the most for you.

Below is a summary of some ingredients and an analysis of what works and what doesn't.

Collagen. When collagen is placed in moisturizers, shampoos and conditioners, it is used to attract moisture. It does this quite well since it can absorb up to thirty times its weight in water. It is a helpful ingredient in hair conditioners because it can penetrate damaged hair. Collagen applied to the skin, however, will have no effect on your skin's own collagen development. The size of the collagen molecule prevents it from being able to penetrate through your skin.

By contrast, injectable collagen is processed as a filler substance that can be injected beneath the surface of the skin. It improves the appearance of wrinkles and scars. People with beef allergies will generally have an adverse reaction to injected collagen and may react to its application on the skin.

Keratin is used as an ingredient in moisturizers because it attracts water. It works well in nail polishes to improve hardness. It is derived from bovine horn, horse hair, boar bristles and quills. It will not affect your skin's keratin production, but is effective at keeping skin moist.

Elastin binds well with water and thus may allow for better moisturizing. It will do nothing to affect or improve your skin's own elastin.

Hyaluronic acid works well as a water binder when applied topically. It can facilitate the penetration of other substances through the skin. It is of animal origin: calf connective tissue, umbilical cords and fluids around the joints.

Placenta. The organ that provides nutrients to the fetus is touted as an accelerator of cellular mitosis, an enhancer of blood circulation and a stimulator of cell metabolism. There is no proof that it does any of these things. It is a complex mixture of proteins. Cow placentas are the most common source. There is no evidence that it will help remove wrinkles. It is generally considered nontoxic. According to the FDA, any product claiming to contain placental extract may be considered misbranded if the extract is made of placentas from which the hormones and other biologically active substances were removed.

Liposomes. Cosmetic companies claim that these microscopic sacs allow for the more efficient penetration of a cream's active ingredients. This allows a sustained release of water-soluble chemicals and other water-binding agents. Liposomes do what they claim. The real issue is whether the ingredients within the liposome are good, and this varies from product to product.

There are hundreds of other ingredients and claims. The list above merely demonstrates that if an ingredient is in a cosmetic, its effectiveness usually boils down to moisturizing or facilitating moisturizing. Paying top dollar for one of these ingredients is a waste of money. While the raw materials may be expensive to obtain and process, that doesn't mean there is any benefit or value to you. It is easy to fall under a *sell spell* and believe that if a product has the same things in it that your skin does, it has to be good for you. Bear in mind that your skin is a complex organ just like your heart or brain. You can't just add more of its constituents to make it work better.

Many cosmetic companies have responded to the cry for oil-free products from women who are prone to breakouts. Moisturizers and foundations contain the most *oil-free* claims. I never tell my patients that they must use oil-free products, especially if they have found a product that is compatible with their skin. If you definitely don't want to use a product with oil, however, beware of ingredients such as glycel tirbehenate, lard, lanolin, carnauba, ozokerite, petrolatum, squalene and mono- or diglycerides. They are just other words for oils. Recent research has suggested, however, that oil may not be so bad after all. Dr. Albert Kligman at the University of Pennsylvania performed a study with twenty adolescents who used petroleum cream or a cream containing only 30 percent petroleum. Amazingly, in both groups there was a slight decrease in the number of blackheads. Dr. Kligman believes that blackheads aren't necessarily produced by oil placed on the skin. In fact, some of the worst blackhead-causing ingredients contain no oil whatsoever. Furthermore, using the right kind of moisturizer actually can help clear acne.

Far more important than oil-free is the label *noncomedogenic* or *nonacnegenic,* meaning that the product doesn't cause blackheads or acne. But even this label isn't perfect. Have you ever wondered how cosmetic companies come to the conclusion that their product doesn't cause pimples? Sometimes they apply the moisturizer or makeup to the inside of rabbits' ears and see what happens. Besides the obvious flaw (a rabbit's ears aren't exactly like human facial skin), the inside of the animal's skin is often not looked at microscopically to determine whether tiny blackheads were starting to develop. Another testing method is to apply the material to the backs of men. Obviously, there's a big difference between that area and the cheek of a thirty-two-year-old woman who has hormonally-related acne problems.

Skin Do's and Don'ts

Spending a few dollars for a jar of collagen-enriched cream is one thing. Using other products that may actually be harmful to your skin or general health is another. There are just some things you should not put anywhere near your skin (unless otherwise authorized by your physician). Here are the no-no's:

Hydrogen peroxide or products containing hydrogen peroxide. Hydrogen peroxide can interfere with the skin's healing process. It has no place in the cleansing of wounds or any type of skin care whatsoever. Clean minor cuts and abrasions with saline instead.

Coal tar. On a purely cosmetic level, coal tars can discolor light hair.

Bubble bath. It can irritate mucous membranes and dry even the heartiest skin.

Dyes or coloring agents. Be judicious in your use of anything with these products. Of course, this is often unavoidable if you are looking for a product such as lipstick, blush and so forth. You do not need dyes in body lotions, hand cream, shampoos or moisturizers, so avoid them. Instead, use brands that do not use dyes or coloring agents, such as Aubrey Organics (800-282-7394 or http://www.aubrey-organics.com).

KathonGC. Don't use—or at least try to avoid—cosmetics, soaps or liquid soaps containing this ingredient, also known as octhilinone, methylisothiazolinone or methylchloroisothiazolinone. This preservative is well known for causing sensitization. More current research shows that it has cancer-causing potential. European countries have directed that the concentration of KathonGC in cosmetics be reduced from thirty parts per million to fifteen. In the United States, the Cosmetic Ingredient Review Board expert panel concluded that KathonGC may be used safely in "rinse-off" products or "leave-on" products in specified concentrations. But other researchers consider this chemical dangerous. Again, this product is ubiquitous and may be impossible to avoid completely. Avoid using any product with KathonGC that is a "stay-on" product.

Ethanolamines, monoethanolamine, diethanolamine and triethanolamine. These are found in soaps and detergents. Also known as ETA, this chemical has been suspected of causing liver cancer.

When buying cosmetics, keep these helpful tips in mind:

- Use well-known name brands. They do not need to be expensive department store products but should be brand names that are familiar to you. Zoe Draelos, M.D., a dermatologist at the Bowman Gray School of Medicine, advises her professional peers to recommend skin care products that have been on the market for at least a year and will remain on the market for the long term. Dr. Draelos also cautions consumers against using products that are marketed only for intrastate or professional salon use since the FDA has jurisdiction only over products distributed between states.
- Keep track of what you are using. In the event that you have a bad reaction (or even a good one!), it's important to know what caused it.
- The fewer ingredients, the better. Dr. Draelos recommends selecting products with less than ten substances to avoid allergic reactions.
- If you plan to see a dermatologist, bring your cosmetics or moisturizer to his or her office for an evaluation.
- Speak to a manager about the store's return policy. Tell the manager you are trying the product for the first time and would like to be able to return the unused portion for an exchange or credit.
- Higher-priced items don't mean you will get more from the product. This is true when you consider that the two most expensive items in a product are fragrance and packaging, neither of which do a thing for your skin.

Safe Cosmetics, Healthy Skin

How much makeup do you own? Of that amount, how much do you use every day? If you're like most people, you probably have six or seven items that are your favorites. The rest sit in a drawer or box collecting dust because they are the wrong colors, have irritating ingredients or are too difficult to apply. Perhaps you were pressured into buying something you didn't need by a strong sales pitch or by a magazine ad. Maybe you believed (or hoped) you could look like the model wearing a particular brand of lipstick or blush. Buying makeup is often an impulsive act. Wearing it to your best advantage, however, requires skill and planning.

In ancient times, women didn't have to worry about learning to apply their own makeup. Young servants applied cosmetics to the ladies of the Roman Empire under the supervision of a woman called the *ornatrix,* an in-house makeup expert. Fads in makeup are nothing new, either. When King Louis IX sprayed a mouthful of red wine over the exposed bosom of a dinner guest, a delicate pink tint developed. Soon commercial products appeared to satisfy the rage for rose-colored breasts. The Hindus used betel nuts to darken not just lips but teeth. Vermilion and other colors were mixed with waxes for facial designations of caste.

Today teenagers agonize over a single pimple and use concealers to cover the problem. In the 1600s women covered the permanent facial scars left by smallpox with a "beauty patch," a small silk or velvet ornament often shaped like the moon or stars.

Cosmetics and perfumes were confined to the upper class and considered a status symbol until around the turn of the century. With the Industrial Revolution cosmetics became affordable to almost everyone. By the 1920s these "little luxuries" were available in American drugstores and quickly became household items. Everyone could afford to look beautiful.

Fads in fashion come and go, but maintaining clear, healthy skin is always in style. How you use and maintain your makeup can have an impact on your skin as much as any new shade of lipstick or blush.

Hypoallergenic

Is the label "hypoallergenic" a guarantee that the makeup, cream or lotion won't cause your skin any problems? No. It merely implies that the product is less likely to cause allergic reactions. There is no standardized test or method to back up this claim. Some companies do testing on their

own; others omit perfumes and fragrances. Other labels such as "dermatologist tested" or "allergy tested" also offer no guarantee that a product
won't cause reactions.

The FDA tried to publish regulations defining hypoallergenic in
1975 and require companies to submit information substantiating their
hypoallergenic labels. ALMAY and CLINIQUE challenged the proposed regulations and after several court appeals, they were able to defeat the FDA's
efforts.

"Natural" is another word that is often placed on a cosmetics
label. Although a company may use plant extracts or herbs in a product,
the base formulas are often the same as in conventional products. Likewise, "no animal testing" means that the company selling the product
didn't test it on animals. In many cases, however, the ingredients in the
product have been tested on animals at some prior time by another
company.

SAFETY FIRST

Cosmetics can cause infections when products become contaminated or are misused. Homemade or off-brand cosmetics may not contain
important preservatives to prevent the growth of micro-organisms.

Here are some general precautions for using cosmetics safely:

- Do not use open samples at cosmetic counters. In one survey of
  makeup counter samples in department stores, more than 5 percent were infected with fungus and other contaminants. Beware
  of having a makeover in a department store. If you do so, insist
  that the applicators used are fresh disposable ones.
- Discard any makeup that smells rancid or has lost its consistency.
- Wash hands before applying cosmetics.
- Wipe off containers with a damp cloth if they become dusty or
  dirty.
- Discard eye cosmetics after six months and mascara after three
  months.
- Use fresh tap or distilled bottled water to dampen eye shadow.
  Never add liquid to bring a product back to its original consis-
  tency. Adding other liquids can introduce bacteria.

- Do not use eye makeup if you have an eye infection. Throw away all products you were using when you discovered the infection.
- Do not store cosmetics above 85 degrees. Doing so can increase the chances of destroying preservatives that protect against bacteria. They can also lose their original consistency.
- Be careful not to scratch the eye. Do not allow any cosmetic to come in contact with the eye.
- Never line the inside of your eyelid. This can damage your eye.
- Serious infections can occur and may permanently affect vision, especially if the eye is traumatized with infected mascara. So don't apply mascara in a moving car.

Product Suggestions for Your Skin Profile

Now that you have learned about your Skin Profile and the best way to care for your skin, here are some suggestions for foundations, shadow and other cosmetics that may be best for you.

HORMONALLY AND STRESS-REACTIVE SKIN

Foundation. Try BOBBI BROWN OIL FREE FOUNDATION or CLINIQUE STAY TRUE OIL FREE. If you have very oily skin, try ERNO LASZLO NORMALIZING TINTED MAKEUP followed with CONTROLLING FACE POWDER. My only reservation about this product is that it is quite expensive and needs to be mixed prior to use.

Powder. Use COVER GIRL CLARIFYING PRESSED POWDER or CORNSILK PRESSED POWDER.

Eye shadow. Avoid creams, pencils and stick formulations. Use powder shadow. To intensify, add a drop of water to a sponge or brush applicator and then mix into the powder shadow.

Environmentally Sensitive Skin

Foundation. Try Elizabeth Arden Flawless Finish Everyday Makeup SPF 10 or Clinique Sensitive Skin Makeup SPF 15, oil-free, fragrance-free and nonacnegenic.

Eye shadow. Avoid shiny, frosted or iridescent eye shadows. These products contain substances with sharp-edged particles that can produce itching. Use eye shadows with a matte finish instead. Darker eye shadow colors also tend to be more irritating than lighter ones.

Overexposed Skin

Foundation. Try Neostrata Exuviance Skin Caring Foundation SPF 15, Maybelline Natural Defense Makeup with SPF 15 or Lancôme Dual Finish Powder (it works both wet and dry).

Eye shadow. Use matte finish in light, natural colors. Apply moisturizing concealer to eyelids before applying eye shadow to even out the pigment and increase the durability of the shadow.

Hearty Skin

As long as you follow the general precautions, you can use whatever you like.

◼ Relax and Have Fun

Unlike plastic surgery, makeup is cheap and washes off. Don't be afraid to experiment and enjoy yourself. If you make a mistake, don't fret. Ask a friend to help with suggestions, especially someone whose look you admire. Keep up to date by reading beauty columns in magazines. By learning how to improve your looks and remaining interested in what works, you're already on the right track. Remember, however, that no amount of makeup can compensate for skin that is neglected.

I saw a sign on the side of a church the other day that read: "As soon as you feel like you're too old to do something, start doing it." That sounds like good advice for a healthy attitude about life and makeup. Give something new a try. It is absolutely refreshing.

Perhaps you won't look ten years younger after finding the right shade of lipstick, but you just might look ten years prettier. Used carefully, makeup is a confidence booster—and feeling good about yourself is essential for looking and feeling younger.

11

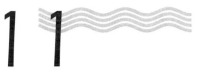

Between Home and the Doctor's Office: Professional Beauty Treatments

My mother called it the "beauty parlor." Today it's a salon, a spa, even a retreat. According to one author, the terms "beauty parlor" and "salon" invoke a time when a woman visited these establishments in order to secure "her place in a round of social visiting, along with shopping, promenading and taking in a matinee." Today our visits may be more streamlined, but even a brief trip to the beauty parlor makes us feel a little special and pampered.

The growth in the number of beauty salons in the United States provides a classic example of a market creating a need rather than a need creating a market. Before the Civil War, American women took care of their own hair. Those with more money had domestic servants brush, set and style their hair. There were no public establishments dedicated to hair care for women. Professional hairdressers as we know them today simply did not exist. Financial and social developments, rather than personal grooming needs, spawned the growth of the beauty parlor. As the economy changed and women found themselves responsible for the financial upkeep of their families, they began to develop careers in hairdressing, cosmetology, manicure and cosmetic sales. Gradually, a beauty culture emerged. Women began to venture outside their homes for the care of their hair, skin and nails.

Today, most salons maintain high levels of sanitation and hygiene, but in days past this wasn't always the case. Before the proper cleansing of hair salon equipment became routine, a certain scalp infection was so commonly associated with contaminated combs that it was called "barber's itch."

The approach to beauty in the hands of aestheticians has become increasingly sophisticated. While you can accomplish many of your skin, hair and nail care goals at home, professional beauty salons provide the finishing touch.

What should you expect from a beauty salon? At a minimum, professional hair stylists, manicurists and aestheticians should provide you with satisfying results in a safe and clean environment. Beyond that, the experience should be relaxing. In the best of all worlds, your beauty parlor should bridge the gap between your at-home skin, nail and hair care routines and the care of a physician or surgeon.

For the most part, the licensing of hairstylists and other beauty professionals is regulated by a state board of health or a professional licensing board. You should always ascertain the credentials of all persons working on you to ensure that they have been properly trained.

DO YOU NEED A FACIAL?

There is no longer one kind of facial; variations now include detoxification, herbal, magnetic, even diamond. Prices can range from $50 to over $300 for one of these treatments. What are you getting for your money and your time?

I can't argue with the fact that a facial is relaxing. It's usually performed in a quiet room to the sound of peaceful New Age music. Gentle strokes glide over your forehead and cheeks. Who can deny the rejuvenating potential of such pampering? When we feel relaxed, we look better. I have seen it time after time on the faces of patients who return from vacations.

Gentle facial massage can stimulate microcirculation and bring oxygen and blood to the tissues and muscles. The immune system gets a boost, sending a surge of "good chemicals" through the body.

Aromatherapy facials provide the added bonus of restorative scents such as lavender, marigold and pine. Facials can provide a temporary boost. I do have three caveats, however, when it comes to facials:

1 *You need relatively good skin for a facial.* I know this sounds a little crazy. After all, don't people get facials because their skin is out of sorts? The truth is that facials make good skin look better. If your skin is not in good shape, you may be asking for trouble. Don't get a facial at a salon if

- You are environmentally sensitive or allergic in general.
- Your skin is sensitive to the touch from sunburn or other irritations.
- Your skin is prone to broken capillaries; facials can aggravate them.
- Your skin has reacted poorly to facials in the past.
- You have been diagnosed with rosacea, or you have an open herpes blister.
- You have more than three or four large, painful pimples; you need to see a dermatologist, not a facialist.

2 *Overzealous claims about the effects of facials on the skin can mislead consumers.* Consider these descriptions:

Aestheticians use a "microdermabrasion" system that sprays crystal powder . . . onto the skin. The powder is vacuumed off the face, exfoliating fine lines.

Your skin will be slightly smoother at best from "microdermabrasion." Fine lines will remain untouched. The benefit will be temporary. Any skin treatment that is deep enough to permanently remove a wrinkle can't be or shouldn't be performed in a beauty parlor.

Clinicians . . . rescue dull facial complexions by brushing warm wax over the face. The heat from the paraffin draws moisture into the skin, leaving it firm and rehydrated.

Perhaps, but the results are temporary at best. I'm skeptical that any facial treatment will actually firm the face.

I have to admit that I had never had a facial until recently. It was relaxing to be on the receiving end of skin treatment. In the long run, however, I was disappointed. After having my face massaged and slathered, I ended up feeling that my skin was greasier than before I started. I also felt that a half-hour of manipulation of the face did more harm than good.

3 *A facial should be gentle.* As I said before, gentle massage of the face does result in a surge of microcirculation, bringing blood and oxygen to the facial tissues. It may also reduce some facial puffiness and swelling if done properly. According to David E. Bank, a dermatologist who specializes in cosmetic procedures, facials are popular because they "feel wonderful" and may transiently smooth the skin. The massage during the facial, however, should be very gentle. Tugging the skin may damage it.

Here are the techniques commonly used in facials:

Steaming. Water is heated and its steam released via a tube onto the face. In some cases the water contains essential oils for an aromatherapy facial. Steaming allegedly deep-cleans the skin and empties the pores of impurities. Gentle steaming may allow for the gentler removal of blackheads and other impurities.

Dr. Bank is skeptical about the benefits of steaming the skin. According to him, steaming causes facial sweating, and sweating won't do anything for blocked pores.

Dry skin may become drier if not properly moisturized while the skin is still damp. Also beware: Steamed skin is fragile and can become abraded if pinched, picked or manipulated too harshly.

You should also be careful about the cleanliness of the water and the steaming machine being used since both can harbor bacteria that has access to your vulnerable skin. Steam that is too hot or too close can damage your skin. If it feels uncomfortable, ask the aesthetician to stop or place the steam farther from your face.

Removal of blackheads. Manipulating the face is a dicey proposition. The gentle removal of blackheads with a properly sterilized instrument can improve the appearance of your skin and keep blemishes from developing. If this is done improperly, however, you run the risk of damaging the skin. Removing blackheads can result in scarring or infection, even from a highly trained professional. If you feel uncomfortable, call a time-out. One of the most important aspects of proper blackhead removal is knowing when to leave a blackhead alone. If it is difficult to remove, it should not be removed.

Scrub or exfoliation. The skin may be scrubbed or sloughed to remove dead skin cells and other debris. Ask the beautician what she is using to scrub the skin. Certain "natural" products can be too rough. Alpha and beta hydroxy acids do a better job at exfoliating the skin than loofahs because they affect the skin at a deeper level.

Application of creams. After the face has been steamed, lotions are applied. Ask the aesthetician what she intends to use on your face. Read the ingredients list. This question is quite significant since the lotion is going to be applied to skin that is damp and has been steamed, allowing maximum absorption and, in some cases, maximum irritation.

Massage. If done correctly, this part of the facial may provide some benefit both in terms of its relaxing effects and its stimulation of blood vessels. The massage should be done gently.

Electrical stimulation. Some salons use an electronic device, which they claim can kill germs. One spa brochure stated the device provided "galvanic ionization" (whatever that means). According to Dr. Bank there is no evidence that electrical stimulation provides any therapeutic benefit.

Microdermabrasion. In recent years, salons have been touting a technique called "microdermabrasion." In essence, it involves the application of micro-pellets to the skin via a tube or other instrument under high pressure. The purpose is to abrade or exfoliate the skin. According to Dr. Bank, your skin may look a bit fresher from microdermabrasion, but considering the cost and time involved, your skin will be better served by using an effective alpha hydroxy acid product at home or seeing a dermatologist for a stronger peel.

Toner or astringent. This may provide a temporary degreasing for oily skin but can also aggravate sensitive skin.

If you decide to get a facial, keep these pointers in mind:

- There is no scientific evidence that a facial will improve wrinkles and other signs of aging on the face.
- Before lying down and closing your eyes, check out the instruments and machines that will be used. Do they look clean to you?
- Do not allow the facialist to "work on" healing blemishes or any open cuts or sores.
- Ask the facialist how she intends to treat your blackheads. Squeezing or removing a closed blackhead may lead to inflammation.
- Regardless of skin type, do not get a facial more than once a month. Once every two months should be enough for most women.
- Although you may expect a little redness after a facial, your face should not be blotchy, irritated or look "picked at" after twelve hours. If this condition persists or becomes worse, consult a dermatologist.

Give Yourself a Facial

If you love the feeling of a facial but can't afford spa visits on a regular basis, you can give yourself one with about the same results. The worst thing about giving yourself a facial is that you can't lie down while doing it. On the upside, you can save money and have better control.

To make the experience more relaxing, you might want to have a friend or partner give you a facial. Make sure your hands or your partner's hands are washed well with an antibacterial soap before the facial.

Try these self-facial techniques:

FOR ACNE-PRONE HORMONALLY REACTIVE OR STRESS-REACTIVE SKIN

- Blot your face gently with a soft tissue.
- Dampen your face with warm water.
- Saturate a cotton ball with brewed yarrow tea and lemon peels. Apply in even strokes over your face. Relax.

- Mix two parts skim milk, one part oatmeal and a teaspoon of kosher salt in a bowl. Apply to your neck and face with a washcloth. Be gentle. No need to scrub. Allow it to sit for five minutes.
- Rinse with warm water followed by cool water.
- Brew peppermint tea, allow it to cool, and apply with soft cloth.
- Rinse with warm water and pat dry.
- For an extra boost, mix half a cup of water, half a cup of vodka and one teaspoon of lemon balm leaves. Store in a tightly sealed jar for one week, then strain. Apply the strained liquid with a cotton ball to your face.

A person with acne-prone skin may not benefit from a salon facial because of the unknown ingredients in the topical products being used and also because manipulation of the skin may stimulate oil glands.

FOR ENVIRONMENTALLY SENSITIVE SKIN

- Allow two cups of plain yogurt (low fat or whole) to sit at room temperature until liquid separates from yogurt. Drain off liquid. You can also strain the yogurt through a cheesecloth. Apply the yogurt to your face. Leave on for five minutes.
- Rinse with cool water.
- Brew chamomile tea, allow to cool. Saturate a soft cotton cloth with the cool tea and place over face like a compress.
- Rinse with cool water.
- Apply an unscented, lanolin-free moisturizing lotion.

FOR OVEREXPOSED OR HEARTY SKIN

- Dampen your face with tepid or warm spring water.
- Boil one tablespoon of fennel in a quart of water and let it steep for several minutes. Reheat the water so that steam rises from it. Remove the water from the heat source and place it in a bowl. Drape a towel over your head and lean over the bowl. Steam your face for two to three minutes. Dampen your face with a cloth that has been immersed in the mixture.
- Pat dry.

- Saturate a cotton ball with extra-light olive or flaxseed oil. Gently apply beginning at your jawline, up the face, under the eyes, to the temple and across the forehead.
- Press a cloth that has been immersed in cool water over your eyes.
- Massage the area between your eyes. Gently pat the area around your eyes.
- After five minutes, rinse with tepid water. Remove excess oil with a damp cloth or cloth diaper.
- Moisturize with recommended night cream.
- Apply cool cloth to the eye area with gentle pats.

PICKY, PICKY, PICKY

Okay, okay, I didn't mention any picking of pimples or blackheads in my at-home facials. I know this won't stop you. Picking one's face can be an overwhelming temptation.

While I want to stick to my admonition against picking your face, I think that I must provide some rules instead of just pretending that you won't do it because I told you not to. Here are the guidelines:

1 Pick only after a shower or after application of a warm, moist compress to the face. The skin needs to be well hydrated. Be careful, however, because your skin will be fragile and easy to abrade.

2 Wash your hands with soap and water before you begin.

3 For whiteheads, gently nick the central portion of the lesion with a small, clean sewing needle. Clean the needle with an alcohol swab and avoid touching the tip of the needle with your hands or placing it on any surface.

4 After nicking the whitehead, *don't squeeze.* Spread the skin around the pimple outward. This allows for the debris to be expressed without damaging the inflamed skin.

5 Gently dab the whitehead with a clean damp cloth.

6 Then leave it alone!

7 For blackheads, begin with Step 1.

8 Gently press the area around the blackhead with the fleshy part of your fingertip, not your fingernail.

9 I don't recommend the use of blackhead extractors by nonprofessionals.

10 Kenet's Law of Face Picking: Look at the clock before you start and stop after five minutes. Do not pick again for at least a week.

Other Salon Treatments

LOOFAH AND SALT SCRUB

This treatment involves the use of a loofah sponge and coarse salt in order to soften the skin. I recommend this only for people with Hearty Skin.

HERBAL WRAPS

Herbal wraps generally involve placing layers of very warm (steamy) cloths on your body. The cloths have been immersed in a mixture of herbs that are supposed to cleanse and purify the body. In some cases the herbal-soaked cloths are layered with rubber covers to insulate the steam. Be forewarned: This treatment can be very hot and may not be suitable for either the claustrophobic or persons with Environmentally Sensitive Skin. A trip to the sauna may provide a similar benefit for less money.

OXYGEN FACIALS

I have heard about a famous television actress who is an avid fan of "oxygen facials." According to some people, she travels with an oxygen tent (hyperbaric oxygen chamber) to look young. It astounds me that someone with unlimited access to top cosmetic care would believe that oxygen applied or surrounding the skin can do anything for her. The definition of an oxygenating facial is a basic facial supplemented with the application of a solution of stabilized oxygen. This may sound impressive, but it will provide no benefit to your skin.

Consider these basic facts: Oxygen is not a vitamin. The U.S. Food and Drug Administration recognizes no substance known as vitamin O. Our atmosphere is 21 percent oxygen. Topical oxygen cannot be delivered into the body via the skin. The skin is supplied with oxygen via the respiratory system. Inhaling pure oxygen may even be unhealthy, especially when it is done over an extended period of time. Equally useless is any kind of oxygen therapy for the face.

COSMETIC TATTOOING

Some women grow tired of putting on and taking off makeup day after day. The idea of permanent makeup in the form of a tattoo sounds like the perfect solution. The most common areas of the face for tattooing are the eyebrows, eyelids and borders of the lips. Before you decide to do this, you should be aware of the potential dangers of this practice.

Tattoo practitioners are often not licensed and may be inexperienced. While a movement is under way in many states to regulate and license persons who provide cosmetic tattoos, there is no federal regulation regarding tattooing and local regulations are uncertain.

The biggest risk for any type of tattooing is hepatitis. According to the American Liver Foundation, tattooing and body piercing may be causative factors in approximately 40 percent of all hepatitis B and C cases with no known source of infection. While this statistic is based on decorative tattooing as opposed to cosmetic tattooing, the numbers are alarming.

According to the Alliance of Professional Tattooists, an organization that educates tattooists in infection-control techniques, these practices should be followed:

● The tattooist should have an autoclave on the premises. An autoclave, which is a device using steam heat, ensures the killing of all bacteria and viruses on instruments.

● Consent forms should be signed before tattooing.

● Immediately before tattooing, the tattooist should wash and dry his or her hands and don medical latex gloves; these should be worn during the entire procedure.

● Needle bars and tubes should be autoclaved after each customer.

● Tissues and other material should be placed in a trash can lined with a plastic bag.

● Used needles and razor blades should be placed in a "sharps" container for disposal.

Even if all these sterilization techniques are employed, you may still be faced with other problems:

- Mistakes are difficult to correct.
- As eyebrows and lips shift downward or change with age, an unwanted cosmetic result may occur.
- Fashion trends change, and the style of eyebrow tattoo or liner selected today may seem outdated tomorrow.
- A condition called tattoo granulomas can occur if your body produces an immune response to the pigment. A granuloma is a firm, raised bump that can be red or inflamed. It is very difficult to treat.
- Cinnabar, used for lip tattoos, is considered one of the most allergenic pigments.

BODY PIERCING

Besides infection, which is the most common complication, there are other serious medical risks associated with body piercing. Allergic skin reactions, large scar formation and swollen lymph nodes can occur. Body piercing has been implicated in the transmission of hepatitis B and C and even HIV. Standardized safety practices are not in effect. Beware.

PROFESSIONAL NAIL CARE

When a professional manicurist is working on your nails, watch what is happening. If she is digging into the cuticle or causing any pain, ask her to stop. Cuticles protect nails from the entrance of water, yeast and bacteria. Because of this vital protective function, you don't want them cut too closely. Ask how the instruments in the salon are cleaned. As mentioned before, the autoclave is the best method of sterilization. If the salon you go to does not use an autoclave, purchase your own set of instruments and either bring them with you or ask if they can be stored in the salon.

Use your intuition and don't be afraid to speak up if you are not satisfied with the way the manicure feels or the way the instruments are handled. If you feel awkward about saying something, just say that the nail is very sensitive.

Don't assume that every manicurist will follow safe and hygienic practices. Take a look around the salon. Is it clean and organized? Does the manicurist look rushed? If you are not happy, don't go to the salon again.

HOT TUBS

While hot tubs per se are not a beauty treatment, I am including them in this chapter because they are often in spas. Hot tubs can present a health hazard to your skin by causing what dermatologists call "pseudomonas folliculitis," a condition characterized by small, red, tender pimples, often on the buttocks and legs. The condition usually resolves spontaneously, but more difficult cases can be treated with topical or systemic antibiotics.

Hot tub folliculitis is associated with tubs that do not maintain adequate chlorine levels. While it may be difficult for you to ascertain whether the necessary chlorine levels within a hot tub are present, do a visual inspection to make sure the tub at least looks clean before stepping into it. Also determine whether the management requires users to shower before entering the tub.

EYELASH DYES

In chapter 10, I briefly discussed the hazards of eyelash dyes. Since professional salons offer this service, I am reiterating my previous admonition. The FDA warns consumers that they should never dye their eyelashes or eyebrows. An allergic reaction can cause swelling, irritation, even blindness. The use of hair dyes for eyebrows and eyelashes is prohibited in beauty salons and other establishments. Having your eyelashes dyed in a salon is absolutely no guarantee of its safety regardless of what any beauty professional may tell you, such as "It's all natural" or "It's from Europe." Remember, arsenic is natural, and Mussolini came from Europe.

12

The Doctor's Office:
The Three C's of a
Good Cosmetic
Physician

You've done all you can. You have followed all my advice. You are looking better and feel comfortable about your skin routine, but you're still craving something more. Perhaps you have a skin condition that is not clearing up. Maybe you are just wondering what a physician can offer that over-the-counter products or even salon treatments can't. Maybe it is time to see the doctor after all. How can you find the right physician who will tend to your skin's needs and leave you feeling medically and emotionally satisfied? Selecting a doctor does not have to be a difficult, time-consuming chore as long as you do a little research and ask the right questions.

Patients looking for professional cosmetic care sometimes fall into the hands of physicians who encourage aggressive procedures that may result in an overdone look. Being unsure about what you want makes you more vulnerable to this unfortunate overreaching. Finding a doctor you can trust will make all the difference.

It is your job to become a skeptical medical consumer. Even very successful "in-control" people can be confused about what they want when it comes to their own face and body.

A Bright Star

She is at the height of her career, although I am certain that many successful years will follow. It is hard to pass a news-stand without seeing her face on the cover of a magazine. Men and women both agree that she is beautiful, some even think flawless. Besides being beautiful, she is a stage and screen actress, admired by many.

One would imagine that a celebrity of her international magnitude would be demanding, high-strung, impatient and completely absorbed with her looks. Her tentativeness, however, was disarming. She wanted something, perhaps plastic surgery, to improve her looks. Could I suggest a procedure? I spent some time just talking to her and told her that she could improve her appearance with careful maintenance, a series of mild face peels and a few minor procedures that I could perform in the office. I plumped out a small scar with saline as a temporary measure to let her "try on" the improvement she would likely get with injectable collagen. I also "zapped" some tiny blood vessels and lightened liver spots on her face with liquid nitrogen. Anything more aggressive would have been a disservice.

After a bit more discussion, I was surprised to learn that she never used sunscreen. I recommended a photo-protective product that was compatible with her complexion and lifestyle. I told her this was the most important service I could offer. Since she lives in a subtropical zone, she could not afford to risk any further exposure without some protection.

When we finished our first session, she looked refreshed, and her skin texture and tone were improved. She has visited me on many other occasions. Regular maintenance visits continue to improve her skin.

I am proud to have helped her understand that plastic surgery was not the right choice for her.

Before discussing specific characteristics to look for in a doctor, you need to know what services each cosmetic-based specialty offers. When a person has cancer, for example, an oncologist is the obvious choice. When a person has a digestive problem, he or she usually sees a gastroenterologist. When it comes to cosmetic care, the choice is not as clear.

Certain physicians are better at one procedure than another. Sometimes this is the result of extended formal training; sometimes the doctor's skill is the product of innate talents or personal interests. Often, the doctor may have had the opportunity to perform the same procedure over and over and has become an expert by virtue of "on-the-job training."

The Cosmetic Specialist

After a physician completes medical school and an additional year as an intern, he or she can obtain a license and begin to practice. No laws prohibit a doctor from offering extremely specialized care—from brain surgery to psychiatry. This is known as a "nonrestricted license." (For practical purposes it is unlikely that a doctor could actually perform brain surgery without the proper postgraduate training since no hospital would grant such a person operating privileges.) This issue is not entirely hypothetical, however. There are cases of obstetricians performing liposuction and internists doing hair transplants. In many cases patients may hardly be aware of their doctor's lack of qualifications.

This lack of regulation places a burden on medical consumers. The following advice can relieve most of that burden and put the odds well in your favor. If you are looking for a doctor to take care of your skin and related cosmetic aging concerns, you should select a specialist from one of these fields, depending on the particular procedure: dermatology, plastic surgery, otorhinolaryngology (ear, nose and throat surgeon), ophthalmology. Seeing any other specialist besides these four may be asking for trouble.

DERMATOLOGIST

A doctor who specializes in the treatment and surgery of the skin, hair and nails is a dermatologist. In order to become a dermatologist, a person must complete four years of medical school, one to three years of medical postgraduate training and three years of a dermatology residency. A typical dermatological practice involves the treatment of acne, psoriasis, allergic skin reactions and hair loss, to name a few conditions.

Some dermatologists concentrate on surgical procedures. The detection and removal of skin cancer, laser surgery and cosmetic procedures are the three major surgical categories within the practice of dermatology. Alan Gaynor, M.D., a dermatologist, summarized the major advancements that dermatologists have contributed to the field of cosmetic surgery: face peels (1882), dermabrasion (1952), hair transplant (1959), laser surgery (1961), liposuction (1977), collagen injections (1979) and tumescent liposuction (1987).

PLASTIC SURGEON

A doctor who specializes in the reconstruction and repair of the external body and face is a plastic surgeon. The word "plastic" is derived from the Greek "plasticos," meaning "to change." Plastic surgeons not only perform cosmetic procedures but attend to the treatment of birth defects such as cleft palates and injuries from traumatic accidents. Many plastic surgeons subspecialize according to their particular interests and background. Surgeons who are more interested in procedures that enhance one's appearance will use the term cosmetic plastic surgeon or aesthetic plastic surgeon. Those who concentrate on repairing injuries or birth defects are known as reconstructive plastic surgeons. It is preferable to choose an aesthetic plastic surgeon for any cosmetic procedure such as a face-lift, nose, eyelid or breast surgery.

A "board-certified" plastic surgeon is one who is certified by the American Board of Plastic Surgery. In order to be certified by this board, a physician must have at least five to six years of approved surgical training that includes a two- to three-year residency in plastic surgery. He or she must also have been in practice for at least two years and pass comprehensive written and oral exams in plastic surgery.

OTORHINOLARYNGOLOGIST (EAR, NOSE AND THROAT SURGEON)

An otorhinolaryngologist, known as an ENT specialist, is a surgeon who concentrates on the ear, nose and throat and treats hearing loss, throat cancers and other related problems. Often an ENT doctor is referred to as a facial cosmetic surgeon since much of his or her training concentrates on the face and the surrounding organs and tissues.

Otorhinolaryngologists who engage in cosmetic procedures are generally members of the American Academy of Facial Plastic and Reconstructive Surgery. In order to qualify in this field, they undergo a head and neck surgery residency with a minimum of one to two years in general surgery. After that, the doctor begins specialty training that lasts four to six years.

Though not required, after residency a few physicians go for further training in a surgery fellowship, a yearlong program during which they train under a senior surgeon.

OPHTHALMOLOGIST

Eyelid surgery to reduce folds, wrinkles and droops of the upper and lower eyelid, also known as blepharoplasty, is often performed by an ophthalmologist. These physicians are trained in both the medical and surgical treatment of the eye. If you are considering cosmetic eye surgery, you should choose a doctor who specializes in eyelid lifts and other appearance-enhancing surgeries as opposed to a physician whose practice focuses on medical surgeries such as cataract removal. An ophthalmologist who subspecializes in cosmetic eye surgery is referred to as an occuplastic surgeon.

Getting Good Advice

How do you start your search for the right doctor?

FAMILY PHYSICIAN

A common starting place is often your family doctor. He or she may have a list of reputable specialists who have proven themselves worthy of special recognition. There are some pros and cons to this approach.

Unlike attorneys, physicians cannot receive "referral fees" from the doctor to whom they send patients. A financial incentive, therefore, does not play a role in the motive for the referral. Bear in mind, however, that referrals may be based on your doctor's friendship or hospital affiliation with another doctor. While referring on the basis of hospital affiliation or friendship is not necessarily a bad thing, it isn't always enough. For the most part, your doctor will recommend you to someone who has proven to be worthy based on reports from satisfied patients. To be on the safe side, ask these questions:

- Does your doctor really know the specialist or is it just a matter of camaraderie?
- How long has your doctor known the specialist?
- Has you doctor seen the results of the specialist's work?
- Does your doctor think you and the specialist will make a good match?

Ask for at least two or three recommendations so that you can make the final decision yourself.

FRIENDS

A second option is to ask your friends, extended family and associates. I think this is a wonderful way to obtain a reliable referral. You are likely to be happy with the doctor since friends usually know one another well enough to understand their needs, preferences and tastes. My only caveat is this: Be a bit wary because some people may recommend doctors just to sound "in the know."

HOSPITAL REFERRAL

A hospital referral source is a list of doctors affiliated with a hospital. Usually, this service is provided over the telephone. The best way to obtain a hospital referral is to call the hospital's main number and ask for the physician referral service. Office hours, areas of specialization, what type of insurance is accepted and other pertinent data are usually available through the service. Overall, the service refers doctors who are associated with the hospital and who undergo a rather stringent selection process. The downside of a hospital referral source is that you are limited to the physicians associated with that particular hospital.

While this may not be my first choice in locating a physician, it is at least a good start. You can be assured that you are in well-trained and qualified hands. University teaching hospitals will probably be the most selective about the physicians that it admits to its staff. Most hospitals generally check credentials, licensures and any complaints against the doctor before allowing him or her to become associated with the hospital. Other helpful resources are Castle Connolly Medical Ltd.'s books, *How to Find the Best Doctors,* which list reputable physicians in New York, Chicago and Florida. For further information, go to <http://www.castleconnolly.com.>

If you want to know more about your doctor's training and whether any disciplinary actions have been taken against him or her, the first place to call is your state's medical society, which handles and processes complaints against physicians. Another resource is a book entitled *10,289 Questionable Doctors.* It lists physicians who have been disciplined by the state or federal government for ethical or other violations. By the way, the number of questionable doctors listed as well as the title of the book change from year to year.

The Three C's

Your goal is to find a doctor who is conservative, competent and compassionate. These essential qualities will create a satisfying relationship between you and your doctor.

CONSERVATISM

Let's start with the concept of a conservative doctor. By conservative I don't mean politically or fiscally conservative. I mean conservative when it comes to cosmetic care. I recommend the least aggressive procedure to achieve a desired result. Most patients appreciate this way of doing things. In addition, I educate my patients about the importance of a healthy skin care routine, which always includes sun protection. The outcome of the best face-lift in the world can be improved by a patient's adherence to the use of three essentials: alpha hydroxy acids, Retin-A and, of course, sunscreen.

A conservative physician will also take the time to evaluate your health status before deciding on any procedure. In other words, the doctor must place your health above any cosmetic concerns. Some of my patients became disappointed when I told them they were not good candidates for a cosmetic procedure because of an underlying medical problem. Most patients have been grateful, however, when I appropriately identified a health problem that would have placed them at too high a risk for surgery.

Cheea

Small-framed, soft-spoken and a bit nervous, Cheea came to my office after being referred by her general practitioner. She spoke in halting English. She had emigrated from Japan ten years earlier and worked her way up from a bank clerk to a manager. Cheea told me she had saved her money in order to afford liposuction to streamline her figure after having three children. On her first visit, we spent some time reviewing her medical history. I explained the procedure to her and informed her about the risks of the surgery. She seemed to understand and was eager to book the appointment as soon as possible.

"Have you ever had a bleeding problem? Any excessive bleeding during surgery, even dental surgery?" I asked.

"No, nothing," she answered.

"Fine," I said. "Let's have some blood tests taken."

When Cheea's blood tests came back, I noticed that a measurement for blood clotting was off by a very small margin. The test tells doctors how efficiently a person's blood can begin to clot and thus stop bleeding. When Cheea returned to my office again, I told her about the results of the test and asked her again if she was aware of this problem. She denied ever being aware that she bled excessively. Because the blood test result was off by only a very small degree and a second blood test turned out to be normal, I agreed to perform the surgery.

Something in the back of my mind still irked me, however. Perhaps it was doctor's intuition or my experience with patients who appear to be not entirely forthcoming. I discussed Cheea's case with a colleague and reviewed her blood tests again, still concerned. The night before the scheduled surgery, I sat Cheea down and asked more questions, this time in a slightly different way.

"Cheea, did you ever have any kind of problem during any kind of medical treatment? Anything at all?"

Cheea furrowed her brow and started thinking. She was anxious to get her liposuction started.

"Well," she said finally, "during a laparoscopy for my uterus, I did bleed for five hours on the operating table, but that was the doctor's fault. He didn't know what he was doing."

It took three visits, two blood tests, over two hours of interviewing and an almost sixth sense on my part to obtain this information. I was shocked but relieved that I had extracted this vital fact. Over her protests, I canceled the procedure.

Consider these factors when evaluating how conservative your doctor's approach is:

- Can the doctor recommend less costly and/or less invasive treatments to accomplish your goals?
- Has your doctor referred you to an internist for a medical evaluation prior to surgery? This is of particular importance if you have a family or personal history of heart problems, if you smoke, if you are over forty or if you have a bleeding abnormality or other systemic disease such as diabetes or high blood pressure.
- Is the doctor comfortable if you choose to seek a second opinion from another doctor?
- Does your doctor take the time to teach you about at-home skin care and sun protection?

COMPETENCE

Competence is a more concrete concept than conservatism or compassion. It speaks to skill, training, judgment and common sense—all vitally important. An Ivy League graduate with years of training is of no benefit to you if he or she can't make important decisions based on both book knowledge and an understanding of human nature.

The best assurance of a physician's competence comes from two major sources: hospital affiliation and board certification.

Ask your doctor about his or her hospital affiliation. Find out if he or she does any teaching at a hospital, even on an unpaid or occasional basis. Generally, a doctor who teaches at a hospital has demonstrated a desire to remain active in academic circles and keep current on developments in the field.

New techniques may be developed after a doctor has finished formal training. Without ongoing study, in a matter of five to seven years a doctor can become out of touch with important developments that can affect your treatment. This is where continuing medical education comes into play. In some cases, doctors are required to obtain a certain number of credits each year to remain certified. In other cases, doctors take courses simply to learn.

Obtaining one's board certification demonstrates a certain level of skill, but even more than that, it shows that the individual wants to attain the highest level of competency and peer approval. Still, board certification is not a guarantee of competency. It's just a starting point.

In some cases, doctors claim to be "board certified," but the "certifying" board is nothing more than an organization that gives a piece of paper to any doctor who pays dues. If you have any doubts about the board affiliation of your doctor, contact the American Board of Medical Specialists and ask about your doctor's credentialing organization. (See listing at the end of this chapter.)

COMPASSION

How much care do you need? Perhaps you are the type who doesn't need a lot of hand holding. Or perhaps you do. One of my patients always requests an extra nurse in the room during a procedure so the nurse can squeeze the patient's hand for reassurance.

Even the most stoic patient needs a doctor who cares. After surgical procedures, follow-up care is essential. You need a doctor who will call on the evening after your surgery. You need someone who is willing to listen to your concerns and with whom you can be honest.

Compassion does not equal love or friendship. You should not seek or expect to be your doctor's best friend. The doctor-patient relationship is at its best when limits are established and carefully maintained. Do not misinterpret professionalism for coldness. You should be comfortable with the way your doctor relates to you. At the same time, the line between caring and being overly familiar should never be crossed.

Consider these issues:

- How do you wish to be addressed? Ms. Smith or Nancy? Let the doctor know your preference.
- Are there members of your family or household who should not be told about your treatment? If so, be sure to tell the doctor.
- Is the doctor doing or saying anything that is making you feel uncomfortable? Speak up.
- Select a doctor who values you and makes you feel comfortable. These characteristics must flow to and from his or her staff as well. Consider the following:
- Is the waiting room comfortable?
- Does the treatment room afford enough privacy?
- Do you feel as if you have your doctor's full attention, or is he or she answering nonurgent phone calls while you are discussing your condition and treatment?
- Are your phone calls to the doctor's office answered promptly?
- Is there a convenient way to reach the doctor after hours?
- Are your questions answered to your satisfaction?
- Does the doctor speak to you with words that you can understand, or does he or she speak in medical jargon?
- By contrast, is the doctor oversimplifying too much?
- Do you understand what the fees are?

Take note of how much time the doctor spends with you. He or she should take a personal interest in your needs. If he or she is rushed and you feel rushed, effective communication can't occur. The doctor should take the time to help you establish your goals. While cosmetic care occurs in a medical setting, it should be as pleasant as possible.

Another important characteristic of a compassionate physician is comprehensive pain control. Your doctor should take an interest in your level of pain tolerance. I have performed liposuction on some patients who haven't required more than local anesthesia and a headset with relaxing music. Others need continuous sedation. My evaluation of a person's pain tolerance and understanding of the potential pain of a procedure is integrated into every plan of care. Pain control matters for smaller procedures as well. When performing relatively minor surgery, I make an effort to eliminate as much discomfort as possible.

Talk to your doctor about pain control, and be sure you feel comfortable about his or her intentions. Remember that it may not be possible to eliminate 100 percent of the pain. Even injecting anesthesia can hurt! Discuss your worries and never be reluctant to ask questions or request further clarification.

A Patient's Responsibility

While determining if your doctor is caring, you should also objectively evaluate your own behavior. You have a responsibility to be a good patient.

- If a question can be answered completely by a nurse or receptionist, don't insist on speaking to the doctor.
- Be on time for your appointments.
- Make a list of questions ahead of time instead of jumping from subject to subject.
- Listen as carefully as possible. If you are too nervous to listen, bring a family member or friend who can be an extra set of ears. At the same time, don't be frightened about asking questions if you are unsure about something.

If you don't like the way you are being treated and aren't satisfied even after expressing your concerns, change doctors.

Remember this: You cannot teach a person to be compassionate. You can very rarely change a person's demeanor and general philosophy just by telling the person that you don't like his or her attitude. The same is true of doctors.

Much of compassion is born of humility. Consider a few of the world's most compassionate heroes—Gandhi, Mother Teresa, Albert

Schweitzer. All of these people were convinced that their contributions to the world were in some way inadequate. This humble attitude is antithetical to many cosmetic physicians, but it is an attribute worth looking for.

I first learned of compassion from my father. As a youth I spent many afternoons in his office. He treated migrant farmers, babies, politicians, domestic workers and even major-league baseball players during spring training. Every person who entered his office was greeted with a welcoming smile. If the patient couldn't pay, my father accepted a basket of locally grown oranges or strawberries.

"When a patient comes in and has something to tell you, sit down," my father advised me. "If you stand, you look as if you are in a rush. It's unfair to stand above the patient. Stay on equal footing."

His advice has allowed me to enter into many wonderful professional relationships with my patients. I think it has also resulted in patients being more satisfied with the cosmetic and medical treatment that I offer them.

Taking the time to find the right doctor is important. The work you put into finding a conservative, competent and compassionate physician will give you a feeling of confidence in your doctor. Satisfaction, security and trust in your physician will be their own rewards.

For information about the board certification of your physician, contact the following organization:

American Board of Medical Specialists
1007 Church Street, Suite 404
Evanston, IL 60201-5913
Phone: 847-491-9091
Fax: 847-328-3596

<http://www.abms.org/addrs/html> This Website has a public education component that can verify the board certification status of any physician certified by the twenty-four ABMS members.

Member boards of the American Board of Medical Specialists include the following:

American Board of Dermatology
Henry Ford Hospital
1 Ford Place
Detroit, MI 48823-6319
Phone: 313-874-1088

American Board of Plastic Surgery
Seven Penn Center, Suite 400
1635 Market Street
Philadelphia, PA 19103-2204
Phone: 215-587-9322

American Board of Otolaryngology
2211 Norfolk, Suite 800
Houston, TX 77098-4044
Phone: 713-528-6200

American Board of Ophthalmology
111 Presidential Boulevard, Suite 241
Bala Cynwyd, PA 19004
Phone: 610-664-1175

13

Be Your Own Dermatologist

Bumps, spots and freckles on your skin can be troubling. I know this based on my encounters with hundreds of people—in elevators, at parties, in theater lines and at beaches. As soon as these casual acquaintances or perfect strangers discover that I am a dermatologist, an urge comes over them to show me something on their skin that utterly confounds them. Women pull up their blouses; otherwise reserved businessmen shimmy to dislodge their shirts from their waistbands; parents disrobe their squirmy children—all in order for me to make a curbside diagnosis.

In this chapter I answer the most common questions that people ask me about their skin.

■ Warts

Common warts, known in medical parlance as verrucae, are firm, rough growths with an irregular surface. They are most frequently found on the hands, feet, face and lower legs. Warts are caused by a viral infection known as the papillomavirus. Scientists have recently discovered that there are more than sixty-five different kinds of viruses that can cause warts. The source of infection is usually human-to-human contact.

Subtle defects in the immune system may make certain people more susceptible to warts, although this phenomenon is not precisely understood. Injured or waterlogged skin provides a good breeding ground for warts. Once granted entrance into the skin, the virus replicates itself and then causes once-normal skin cells to develop into a wart.

Warts can appear on almost any part of the body and are classified into several categories based on their location and shape:

A *plantar wart* is a wart on the sole of the foot that may grow into the thick skin of that area.

A *periungual wart* is found underneath or around the fingernail.

A round, pink, flat-topped wart, called a *flat wart,* is found mainly on the back of the hands, face, neck, wrist and knees. This type of wart is easily spread by shaving over existing warts and infecting other areas as the razor goes over the skin.

A *venereal wart* is a pink, cauliflowerlike growth found on and in genitals and rectum and is sexually transmitted. *Venereal warts must be treated by a doctor. Do not use home remedies.*

TREATMENT

No single type of medical therapy has proven to be 100 percent effective for warts. One of the most challenging aspects of treating warts is getting rid of all the infectious material so that the wart does not regrow. It may look as if all of the wart has been removed, but virus particles that are left behind can replicate and produce yet another wart.

Warts can be treated at home with the use of salicylic acid in such over-the-counter products as TRANS-VER-SAL WART REMOVAL KIT (800-929-9300) or SAL-ACID PLASTERS (800-PEDINOL). To get the most out of the treatment, gently abrade the area before applying the acid. Use a pumice stone or a superfine emery board to slough off any skin that may interfere with penetration of the acid. (Discard the emery board after use. Wash the pumice stone with soap, rinse and air-dry.)

Genital herpes occurs near or on the genital region or the buttocks. The first outbreak of genital herpes is usually the most painful and may be associated with fever, body aches and swollen lymph glands in the groin area. In most cases, recurrences produce fewer blisters, heal more quickly and are without systemic symptoms.

PREVENTION

Since the herpes virus is transmitted by touching, kissing or other sexual contact, it is essential to avoid contact with the lesions. Using condoms is very important as a method of prevention against genital herpes. Abstinence is the only guarantee against transmission during breakouts.

If you have herpes and want to prevent recurrent breakouts, there are some steps you can take. With respect to oral herpes, sun exposure and trauma to the lips and mouth (dental work) can cause a herpes blister to appear. If you notice that dental work triggers an outbreak, consider taking a course of antiviral medication (discussed below) before your dental appointment. Another type of trauma that can cause an outbreak is the irritation that occurs from using tissues to blow your nose. If rubbing your nose seems to trigger breakouts, use the softest tissues available such as PUFFS WITH ALOE. Be careful about sun protection. Use CHAPSTICK LIP BALM ULTRA SPF 30 or NEUTROGENA LIP BALM WITH SPF 15, especially if you plan to be outdoors.

Stress and fatigue can cause both oral and genital herpes to recur. If you discover a connection between your herpes and emotional problems, refer to chapter 6 in this book on Stress-Reactive Skin and try to integrate stress-reduction techniques into your lifestyle.

TREATMENT

Antiviral drugs such as ZOVIRAX and newer compounds such as FAMVIR and VALTREX have provided significant relief for people who suffer from either oral or genital herpes. At the first sign of a herpes outbreak, take the medication per your doctor's orders. These drugs reduce both the severity and the duration of the blistering. The key to effective treatment is starting early. Some patients have reported headaches and diarrhea as side effects of these antivirals, but for most people there are no problems.

Allow the acid to work and don't pick the wart. You run the risk of infecting other areas of your body. Since warts are infectious, avoid touching any warts on another person's body. Wear water shoes, if possible, when swimming in a pool since public pools are a common breeding ground for warts. This is especially important for a child.

Doctors can remove warts by freezing them with dry ice (cryotherapy) or burning them off with a small electrical needle (electrodesiccation), or with a laser.

Sometimes, warts go away on their own. In fact, in studies of children, two-thirds of warts regressed within two years without any treatment.

Folklore and herbal remedies abound in wart treatment. If you are reluctant to use commercially available acids, you might try these home remedies found in *The Illustrated Encyclopedia of Natural Remedies,* by C. Norman Shealy, M.D.:

- Rub a fresh lemon on the wart every day and keep the wart moist with a plaster.
- Squeeze the sap of a dandelion stalk on the wart daily.
- Mix castor oil and baking powder into a paste; apply at night and leave exposed during the day.

Herpes

Herpes simplex, a viral infection, causes blistering eruptions on the skin. There are two kinds of herpes: oral and genital. The first sign of either type is a flat red patch that changes into a blister. After a day or two, the blister breaks open, leaving an open sore. Within eight to nine days the sore crusts over and heals.

People often know when a herpes blister is about to develop because of a tingling and burning sensation on or below the skin before the actual blister appears. Treatment is most effective during this early stage of a breakout.

Oral herpes usually occurs near or on the lips and sometimes the nose. It affects 25 percent to 40 percent of the U.S. population.

Antiviral creams are also available: ZOVIRAX and DENAVIR. They can reduce the pain of a herpes blister and speed healing but are not as effective as pill forms. I recommend them for use along with the pills.

For people who suffer from very frequent outbreaks, ongoing prophylactic therapy is an option. This involves taking antiviral tablets every day. I also recommend a short course of prophylactic therapy during especially stressful times such as final exams or when a herpes outbreak would be very problematic, such as on your honeymoon.

If you want to use home remedies once you have a full-blown outbreak, I recommend DOMEBORO SOLUTION, which can dry out the sores and ease some of the discomfort. Domeboro is an astringent solution available over the counter in drugstores. It should be mixed with water and applied with a soft cloth or paper towel.

For some people, camphor-based products such as BLISTEX or CARMEX can help with the discomfort. Ice placed directly on the blister can reduce swelling and pain.

One expert on the herpes virus, Dr. Kenneth H. Neldner, a dermatologist at Texas Tech University Health Science Center in Lubbock, reports that stress-reduction techniques will not shorten the course of a preexisting outbreak but may be beneficial in avoiding the development of new lesions. Dr. Neldner also reported that some studies have shown that individuals who are deficient in iron, folate, vitamin C or B_{12} improved or thought they had improved by taking supplements.

A very new and experimental treatment for genital herpes blisters is being studied by the Food and Drug Administration. A handheld device called Viratrol delivers a mild electrical current to the site of the cold sore. Studies in China showed that healing time was shortened for people using the machine. Researchers theorize that the current affects the nerve fibers near the basal epithelial cells, creating a hostile environment for the virus.

Developments from Sun Exposure

FRECKLES

Yes, they can be cute, especially on little girls and boys. But my professional training gets in the way, and all I see are signs of sun damage on a person with vulnerable skin. Sun-induced freckles on an adult are associated with a reported fourfold increase in nonmelanoma skin cancer and an even higher risk for melanoma.

The medical term for freckles is ephelides. They are small, flat brown marks that appear on skin that has been exposed to the sun. They are common among persons with blue eyes and red or blond hair. Freckles can be distinguished from age spots in three ways: (1) They appear on young skin, (2) they usually occur in a cluster or sprinkling and (3) they tend to gradually lighten in the absence of sun exposure. Freckles seem to run in families, but you probably didn't need a doctor to tell you that.

Freckles can be lightened but usually not completely removed. An alpha hydroxy acid cream works well if applied on a regular basis and combined with sun avoidance and the use of sunblock. Using Retin-A, available by prescription in combination with an AHA cream, will work even better than one product alone.

I recommend alternating the use of Retin-A and alpha hydroxy acid at night and using a good sunblock during the day. Natural approaches include using lemon juice (which is a fruit acid) on the affected area.

Your dermatologist can lighten freckles by freezing them with liquid nitrogen (dry ice) or using stronger acid peels or a laser.

SOLAR LENTIGO

A splotch of darkened flat skin, often brownish in color, is called a "solar lentigo." The term can be loosely translated as "sun lentil," a rather apt description. In common language it is called a "liver spot" or "age spot." If you are white and over sixty, there is a 90 percent chance that you have one of these on your skin. Your odds go up if you sunburn easily. People with darkly pigmented skin rarely have these spots. Tanning beds are also implicated as causes of solar lentigines.

The presence of solar lentigines on your body should send a message—you've had way too much sun, especially for your skin type. Maybe you think you don't have solar lentigines because there is not a spot in sight. Think again. If you really want to know, go to a dermatologist's office and ask to see your skin under a Wood's Lamp. Then turn out the lights. Look at your face, and you'll see what your skin will look like in ten or twenty years. Sun damage not visible to the naked eye shows up under a Wood's Lamp. All the spots and freckles that will appear in the future can be seen.

Solar lentigines rarely develop into skin cancer.

Solar lentigines will usually not go away by themselves and can enlarge and darken over time. They can be treated with liquid nitrogen or a laser at a doctor's office. Bleaching creams usually don't work.

Seborrheic Keratosis

Dermatologists like to call these little rough stuccolike plaques "sebs." They are so common that most people develop one in their lifetime, and many people develop hundreds. They can appear on any part of the body. When they first appear, they look like flat, sharply demarcated brown marks. As time goes by, they develop an uneven surface and look a bit "warty." Although they are most commonly brown in color, they can also be pink or black. No one is exactly sure why sebs occur. Seborrheic keratoses become more common as we grow older.

The application of liquid nitrogen by a dermatologist is usually the best treatment for sebs.

Skin Tags

Skin tags are small flesh-colored growths that "hang" off the skin. They often appear on the eyelids and underarm. Besides being unattractive, skin tags on the neck can become chafed and irritated by necklaces or collars.

No one knows why skin tags occur, but they can crop up during pregnancy and often disappear after delivery. Skin tags should be removed by a physician. In general, they can be snipped with a surgical scissor and usually do not leave a scar. It's not wise to try to remove the skin tags yourself.

Moles

A mole is a collection of pigment cells. Some people have more moles than others, but most people have at least one. The color of a mole can range from tan to dark brown or even pink. Some are flat; others are raised. A normal mole has a homogenous surface and color, as well as smooth borders. You should examine your skin on a regular basis to determine if any of your moles have changed in size, shape or color. If you notice any changes, see your dermatologist.

Features of a mole that may be dangerous are summarized by the **ABCD** warning signs.

- **A**symmetry: If you were to draw a line down the center of the mole and compare the shape of the two sides, they would be different.
- **B**order irregularity: jagged, uneven edges.
- **C**olor: variation within the mole or changing color.
- **D**iameter: greater than 6 millimeters (larger than a pencil eraser).

Large Pores

The term "large pores" is truly subjective. Get anyone in front of a good mirror and a bright overhead light, and nine times out of ten he or she will recoil at the size of his or her pores.

Patients always ask me if there is any way to shrink, decrease or just get rid of facial pores. We all want that baby skin look—smooth as porcelain and without a pore in sight. The problem is, adults have bigger pores than babies no matter what they do. At puberty, pores increase in size as sex hormones stimulate oil production and sebaceous glands develop.

Pores also grow in size, or at least become more noticeable, when they hold oil and accumulate dead skin cells. Pulling, squeezing and tugging the skin also can increase pore size.

Nothing will really change your pore size, which is often genetically determined. Large pores are also the result of anatomic variation. For example, the central face tends to have large pores while the sides of the face have smaller ones.

Gentle exfoliation and the use of alpha hydroxy or salicylic acid cleansers and lotions can reduce the appearance of large pores. Retin-A can also help, especially if you have blackheads that make your pores look bigger. Use products that work gently over time for the best results.

You can prevent your pores from becoming even larger by being diligent about avoiding sun exposure and using sunscreen. Sun damage to the skin is implicated in the development of both blackheads and large pores.

The use of blackhead-reducing strips such as BIORÉ PORE PERFECT DEEP CLEANSING STRIPS is now the rage for removing blackheads. The strips are a far better alternative than manual extraction, which can leave the skin irritated and the pore larger. However, these strips contain potentially irritating ingredients and should not be used by people with sensitive skin. Furthermore, they should not be used by people using Retin-A or Accutane, or anyone who has face peels or a skin condition such as rosacea or eczema.

Apply concealer to the most troublesome pores. Let the concealer set for two minutes, then spread liquid moisturizer over the entire face and set with loose powder.

Blisters

Blisters develop when the top layer of the skin (epidermis) and the second layer (dermis) separate from each other and fill with fluid. As most people know, this can occur with any burn or friction. Blisters are best left alone. They actually heal better that way. If absolutely necessary, the fluid can be drained by introducing a sterile needle to the blister. Do not remove the loose skin after drainage. Loose skin is the best "bandage" for the underlying wound. BACITRACIN OINTMENT, available over the counter, can be applied once or twice a day. You can also soak the blister in DOMEBORO'S SOLUTION to dry it up.

The most effective commonsense prevention tip for foot blisters is to wear comfortable shoes. If you are "breaking in" a new pair of shoes, wear them for only one or two hours at a time if possible. Bring along an older, more comfortable pair to wear in between.

A recent study by the United States Army found that using deodorant such as DRY IDEA on your feet can prevent blisters during long walks.

Corns and Calluses

Corns and calluses develop from skin under friction. Tight shoes, working with tools or weight lifting are common causes of calluses. Corns are painful calluses on the joints of your toes.

To treat calluses, soak the area in warm water and then rub down the callus with a pumice stone. Natural remedies include placing your feet in a basin with four tablespoons of crushed mustard seeds and warm water.

Be careful when using a blade or razor to pare down a callus. This is best done by a physician to avoid injury to tender underlying skin.

Stretch Marks

Stretch marks are fractured collagen. Skin under stress from pregnancy, weight gain or muscle enlargement may develop stretch marks, also known in medical language as striae. In fact, 90 percent of pregnant women develop at least some kind of stretch marks. In pregnancy, stretch marks generally appear over the abdomen, hips and buttocks. While moisturizing creams and lotions such as cocoa butter may ease some of the dryness associated with pregnancy, no preventive treatment seems particularly helpful for stretch marks. No one knows why they appear, although the most widely accepted theory is that increased hormonal activity along with the increased size of various parts of the body may be responsible.

Stretch marks do fade over time. Take care to avoid exposing this area to the sun. Although no one treatment has been proven to be completely effective for stretch marks, you may want to try some of these approaches: alpha hydroxy acids, Retin-A, lasers or massage.

Spider Veins

A spider vein, also known as a telangiectasis, develops as a result of a structural abnormality within the veins. Larger dilated veins are referred to as "varicosities" or "varicose veins." Each vein has a valve that controls the flow of blood. If the valve does not work properly, it may allow blood to overfill a vein, causing the vein to become swollen and in some cases visible. Besides this structural problem, spider veins also crop up as the result of pregnancy when blood volume increases and places enormous pressure on the venous system.

Spider veins on the face can be removed by electrocauterization, a method whereby a fine electrified needle zaps the vessels and causes them to collapse. Lasers work even better by closing off the vessel. Small veins on the legs can be treated with a laser or an injection of saline solution (sclerotherapy), irritating the lining of the vessel and causing it to close off. Larger leg veins are treated with either sclerotherapy or surgery to remove the vein. To increase the likelihood of success of this therapy, use compression stockings immediately after your treatments or super-strong support hose such as BEIERSDORF JOBST (800-537-1063) or SIGVARIS COMPRESSION PANTYHOSE (800-322-7744).

You may not be able to control the development of spider veins, but you can take the following precautions to reduce your chances:

- Wear support hose, especially if you have a job that requires extensive standing or walking.
- Elevate your legs as much as possible after work.
- Don't smoke.
- To prevent facial spider veins, avoid sun exposure since ultraviolet radiation may play a role in the dilation of the vein itself.

Cellulite

It's the kind of fat that almost all women dread. Puckered, dimply skin, otherwise known as cellulite, on the thighs, hips and buttocks remains a mystery on many levels. Where does it come from? Why can even thin people have it? And the most important question of all: How can we get rid of it forever?

The honest answer is that nobody knows. And anyone who promises to make cellulite disappear is more interested in making your money disappear than anything else. This is what we know to be scientifically true:

- Up to 85 percent of postadolescent women have some cellulite on their bodies. It does not appear in women until after puberty.
- It very rarely appears in men.
- It is not related to obesity.

One interesting but as yet unproven theory about the origins of cellulite suggests that subcutaneous fat pokes through defects in the dermis. These defects occur as a result of an inflammatory process which activates enzymes that damage collagen and elastin.

CELLULITE TREATMENT OPTIONS

Losing weight. In some situations, losing weight might reduce the appearance of cellulite if you are lucky enough to shed inches in areas where cellulite typically appears. In general, however, losing weight is not the complete answer to the disappearance of cellulite.

Liposuction. Usually, liposuction does not help reduce cellulite and in some cases may even create a more rippled appearance on the skin.

Creams and lotions. A few years ago, cellulite creams were the rage. Everyone was massaging their thighs with salves that promised smoother skin. The furor has died down since the promises never really lived up to reality. The first category of creams is known as xanthines; these creams can contain caffeine and aminophylline. While xanthines do contain properties that can break up fat, the problem was the failure of these creams to reach subcutaneous tissue in adequate concentrations and for enough time. If they could actually make a difference, these creams would be classified as a drug and require a prescription, which they do not.

Exercise. While exercise may provide some benefit, it is not a guaranteed way to lose cellulite.

Herbals. Naturopaths recommend massaging the area with juniper-infused oil. Using a blend of rosemary, geranium, grapefruit and cypress in a massage and skin lotion may stimulate the tissues and reduce the appearance of cellulite. An infusion of ginger or chewing fresh ginger daily is also supposed to be beneficial in reducing cellulite.

Skin kneading (endermologie). In this process, a massage machine rolls and unrolls the skin by using suction. Patients usually receive fifteen-minute sessions twice weekly for about two months. After that, maintenance treatments are recommended once a month. According to one study, endermologie is a "mildly effective method for fat mobilization and body contouring." An appropriate candidate for endermologie is a woman under fifty-five with cellulite and small saddlebags who has the time to devote to these treatments.

Cysts

Common cysts result from the proliferation of skin cells that are trapped under the skin and then become enclosed in a saclike structure. Cysts are usually dome-shaped and protrude from the skin. The growth can usually move when manipulated. Cysts are usually not sore or tender.

Some cysts have a small hole in the center that represents a plugged follicle. By applying gentle pressure, a cheeselike material can be expressed through this hole. Cysts commonly appear on the face, neck, chest and upper back where sebaceous glands are numerous.

If you have a cyst and find it annoying or unsightly, it can be surgically removed by a physician. Do not manipulate a cyst yourself since this may lead to a rupture or infection. If this occurs, apply frequent hot compresses to the area.

Another type of cyst, called "milia," appear as minute, superficial, pearly white round growths that arise most commonly on the face, especially the eyelids and cheeks. Milia can be extracted by a physician with a scalpel or blackhead extractor.

If you are concerned about any skin condition or new growth on your body, you should consult a dermatologist. This is especially true if you are concerned about a changing mole. If you are at an increased risk for skin cancer (light complexion, blistering sunburns as a child, family history of skin cancer), you should see a dermatologist for a yearly skin check.

And if you absolutely must, go to a party where you know a dermatologist will be attending. Find a well-lit room, wear loose clothing and ask him or her to tell you what that spot really is!

14

The Natural Way to Beauty

Some of my patients can't take drugs for a number of reasons, such as pregnancy, a propensity for serious side effects, allergies or a limited budget. Others simply don't like the idea of taking drugs. For people with a chronic skin disease such as eczema or psoriasis, conventional medical treatments often don't work. When I look for a way to alleviate skin problems without causing new ones, natural remedies are sometimes the answer.

Despite years of intensive study, there is still a lot we don't know about our skin. Why is it that some people never develop skin cancer even though they spend many hours in the sun? How can we stop the skin from aging? Why do skin diseases like psoriasis and eczema sometimes resist treatment? The bottom line is that traditional medical treatments have their limitations. Effective medications can often present a host of side effects. Patients develop resistance to certain drugs, requiring them to take more and more for relief. How can we deal with these problems? Looking to herbal, nontraditional remedies is one answer. Natural ingredients play a role in healthy skin and the antiaging process. They always have. Moreover, natural approaches can enhance the benefits of traditional medicine.

Before delving into a discussion of natural and alternative medicine, I want to tell you that I am neither an herbalist nor an alternative medicine practitioner. I am, however, someone who believes that sometimes the best medicine is simply to wait for our bodies to heal themselves. Rashes retreat, scars fade and some infections resolve without any intervention—proof of our natural systems at work. Rest and patience sometimes heal us as much as pharmaceuticals.

I have also had the good fortune to learn about alternative medicine from an enlightened family member. Stacia, my sister, practiced pediatrics in California after graduating from Tufts Medical School in Boston. Over time she grew increasingly disillusioned by the overuse of antibiotics for common childhood ear infections and the lack of knowledge about prevention and nutrition. She described seeing many young patients whose illnesses could have been avoided if more attention had been paid to staying well. Stacia decided to open an alternative pediatric practice. She studied alternative medicine and herbal therapies. Her enthusiasm and clear thinking have done much to persuade me that natural cures have a place in the care of patients.

Throughout this book I have made an effort to point out safe home remedies or simple over-the-counter products that can help you look better and younger. In this chapter I will tell you about alternate routes to healthier, better skin.

Self-Healing

One of the most effective natural approaches is simply allowing the body to heal itself. Our skin is quite a marvelous and resilient organ. Consider all the scrapes and cuts that your skin has endured throughout a lifetime and how most of them have mended with little more than soap and water and perhaps a bandage. In more serious cases you may have required a stitch or two. With a little time the skin looks like itself again. Our skin also performs amazingly well under assault by the sun. It is continually attempting to repair the injury.

"Healing by secondary intention" is a medical phrase used by dermatologists to describe how wounds heal by themselves. In certain areas of the body, such as the ear and the side of the nose, healing by secondary intention is a preferred modality of treatment. That's because these areas of the body heal with fewer scars when left alone.

Conditions such as hives, minor burns including sunburns, and mild skin infections can resolve without medicine. Keeping our bodies healthy and our immune system in good shape allows our skin to recover from these problems.

What Does the Natural Approach Offer?

The term natural or alternative medicine has a multitude of definitions and can embrace a wide spectrum of practices. Some of the modalities—such as acupuncture, mind/body relaxation and meditation—have received validation by mainstream medicine. Others are utterly devoid of effectiveness—such as iridology (gauging a person's general health by the color of the iris). Many have yet to be proven or disproven.

When I use the term alternative medicine, I am talking about these principles: an emphasis on diet and lifestyle as a means to health, preventive measures such as early detection and treatment of disease, a focus on the whole patient rather than individual parts of the patient and a reliance on the body's power to heal itself.

The Basic Natural Remedies

Not all natural treatments come in the form of herbs or vitamins. In fact, simple approaches can do wonders.

Ice. To reduce swelling, soreness, redness or inflammation, use ice in a plastic bag. When blemishes become inflamed, either from irritating medications or from too much manipulation, an ice pack can help to make the lesions less noticeable.

Ice cubes. They are great itch relievers. The nerve pathway that conducts the sensation of itchiness also conducts temperature. By numbing the area with cold, you can effectively put an itch on hold.

Warm water. Before using antibiotics or surgery to treat infections under the skin, I recommend to my patients that they use warm water soaks. This simple technique is especially effective for bacterial infections of the fingernail and toenail. Simply immerse the nail in a basin or glass of hot but not boiling water for three to four minutes several times a day.

Salt water. An excellent gargle for canker sores and minor gum irritations, salt water reduces swelling in these areas.

Vaseline and Aquaphor. To promote wound healing, place a dab of Vaseline or Aquaphor over the affected area. Scientific studies have shown that Vaseline helps to heal minor wounds faster than those exposed to air.

Domeboro Solution. This over-the-counter product provides comfort for cold sores, minor infections and poison ivy. It dries up blistered and other "weepy" skin problems.

Milk. The anti-inflammatory properties of milk can ease dry skin. To treat sunburn and poison ivy, apply a whole-milk–soaked washcloth to the affected area for about fifteen minutes. For sunburned faces, cool yogurt can provide relief.

Humidifiers. During winter months, low moisture in the atmosphere can make skin suffer. Using a humidifier can provide extra moisture. This is especially helpful for people who suffer with eczema.

Bedsheets. Soaked in cool water, a wet bedsheet draped over inflamed skin provides comfort for those bothered by itchy psoriasis or sunburn.

Distraction. Whether it's meditation, shopping or a good laugh, distracting yourself from (not ignoring) itchy skin, a sudden acne breakout or other minor skin problems allows your body to heal.

When to Use Alternative Methods

An essential part of utilizing alternative practices is knowing which conditions may respond to them and which conditions require traditional therapy. It is naive to expect that all of our ailments will disappear with the use of an herb. In fact, certain skin disorders are best treated with standard medical therapy because the side effects are minimal and the overall effectiveness is quite high. At the risk of oversimplifying the issue, one could say that chronic skin problems may be better suited to the use of alternative medicine than acute conditions. Acute medical conditions are sudden in onset—a broken leg, for example, or a skin problem such as cellulitis—a bacterial infection of the deep skin tissue. Chronic problems, which wax and wane and are more long-standing, include eczema and psoriasis.

For some skin conditions the decision to use traditional or nontraditional methods depends on one's philosophical bent. Impetigo, a superficial infection often seen around the mouth, responds well to antibiotics. Herbal remedies may also work, though less quickly.

Skin cancers such as basal cell carcinoma, squamous cell carcinoma and melanoma must be treated with surgical removal to ensure that the condition does not spread or worsen. Overall, surgery involves a relatively low risk and offers a very good chance of cure. Alternative medicine should be used only as an adjunct in this setting.

In terms of preventing skin cancers as well as premature aging of the skin, nothing works better than sun avoidance, covering up and applying sunscreen. No natural products can substitute for these commonsense precautions.

Acne provides an excellent example of a medical condition that falls somewhere in the middle. It can be treated with strong medications such as ACCUTANE, but even this drug does not guarantee results and may have severe side effects. Herbal remedies and dietary supplements are by no means a panacea for acne, but they can decrease inflammation and may be gentler on the skin.

I have therefore limited my suggestions for alternative therapy to those conditions that qualify under these two basic criteria: (1) limited effective treatment in traditional therapy, and (2) an alternative method that will do little harm.

ARE YOU THE TYPE?

An important issue regarding the use of herbal and other types of alternative medicine concerns your own expectations and value system. Most herbal remedies require patience. The benefit may appear only after a steady and committed regimen. Consider, for example, how one takes care of a headache. Pop two aspirins and relief often comes within fifteen minutes. Using an ice compress over the affected area and resting may provide some easing of symptoms, but not as quickly.

To benefit from herbal and alternative remedies, you should be willing to experiment a bit. You need to have an open mind about the possibilities of herbal healing, and become an avid but critical reader of journals and reliable sources of information that explain the proper way to deal with herbs. At the same time, you should not be too naive or gullible. The unregulated world of supplements is full of overblown promises that can mislead the unsuspecting person. "Natural" is not a synonym for "safe" or "effective."

Natural remedies provide a relatively safe way to relieve our problems. When I say "relatively safe," I mean just that. In this chapter I will explain how to make sure that the herbs and other ingredients you choose to sample are used safely. I will also offer advice on a sensible and balanced approach to "natural beauty."

Antioxidants: The Free Radical Scavengers

According to the latest theory on aging, chemical fragments called free radicals attack cells throughout our bodies, pierce their membranes and damage their DNA. These assaults occur on a daily basis and affect every organ in the body, including the skin. Free radicals are therefore implicated in the aging process. Our bodies are bombarded with free radicals via cigarette smoke, chemicals, ultraviolet radiation and even some kinds of food. In response to the free radicals' destructive process, our body calls forth antioxidants. These powerful molecules attempt to limit the damage done by free radicals. According to researchers, our body is able to undo at least 99 percent of the damage from free radicals. This still leaves an accumulation of cellular damage that needs to be repaired. Researchers now believe that we may be able to slow down the effects of free radical damage with antioxidants. Antioxidants in abundant quantities in certain fruits and vegetables as well as antioxidant supplements help fight free radical damage to the skin and may speed healing. They slow down damage to the cells and, some theorize, will keep you looking younger, too.

Ultraviolet radiation is the archenemy of skin, but it plays an important role in the growth of plants and other food sources. Without the sun, life could not exist. Scientists theorize that antioxidants developed evolutionarily as a means of protection against ultraviolet damage during photosynthesis. Thus, plants are a rich source of antioxidants. Eating fruits and vegetables, therefore, provides our bodies with protection against the ravages of disease and time. Our own skin also harbors antioxidants as a means of natural protection.

Antioxidants and nutritional supplementation show promise in other areas of treating skin disease. In a recent study, doctors found that treating nutritional deficiencies of vitamin C, folic acid, iron and vitamin B_{12} could halt the spread of vitiligo, a disorder characterized by a loss of pigment over certain areas of the body.

Having discussed the basics of free radical damage within our body, I would like to turn to exciting developments in the area of antioxidants and skin care. The most powerful antioxidants for our bodies in general happen to be the best supplements for our skin as well. They are vitamins A, E, C and B and essential fatty acids such as evening primrose or flaxseed oil.

VITAMIN A, ALSO KNOWN AS BETA-CAROTENE AND RETINOL

Vitamin A is probably the most important vitamin with respect to the skin, both in traditional and nontraditional medicine. The best example of its use in traditional dermatology is Retin-A, Accutane and other retinoid-based drugs. Retinol is also very important in vision; its name was derived from its beneficial effects on the retina. When there is not enough vitamin A in the body, night blindness can occur. Yellow and orange fruits and vegetables contain carotene, which converts to vitamin A. Our body's absorption of carotene and conversion to vitamin A from these sources can be compromised by the use of alcohol or an excessive iron intake or if we have a vitamin E deficiency.

Vitamin A helps skin cells develop normally and gives the skin its structural integrity. Dry, bumpy skin, especially on the backs of the arms, may be the result of a vitamin A deficiency.

Along with adequate protein intake, vitamin A produces healthy hair and nails. The antioxidant effect of vitamin A is well known. It stimulates immune activity, helps to fight off infections and reduces the damage caused by environmental pollutants.

Research shows that 25 percent of people in the United States are deficient in this vitamin. Note, however, that since vitamin A is stored in the body and not readily secreted, toxicity may occur from mildly increased doses over an extended period of time, such as a month or two. Most people should take an oral supplement of 5,000 IU daily of vitamin A or 17,000 IU of beta carotene daily.

Retinol cream, although weaker than Retin-A–type products, can smooth sun-damaged skin by reducing fine lines and skin discolorations. Retinol has antioxidant effects on the dermis and epidermis, and increases cellular turnover. It also helps new cells retain moisture more effectively. Use retinol at night and be sure to wear adequate sunscreen during the day since Retinol may increase your skin's sensitivity to the sun. Recommended products are TxSYSTEMS by Medicis Pharmaceutical Corporation, and RETINOL-15 and RETINOL-30 by Sothys, USA (must be obtained through a physician or a skin care professional). Products with 0.25 percent to 1 percent are usually tolerated by normal skin.

Food sources for carotenes include green leafy vegetables and yellow-orange vegetables and fruits such as carrots, apricots, mangoes, pumpkins, yams and squash.

Warning

Pregnant women or women contemplating pregnancy should consult their physician regarding the use of vitamin A. Birth defects have been linked to the use of certain amounts of vitamin A during pregnancy.

VITAMIN E

Vitamin E is probably the best-documented nutritional antioxidant in dermatology. D-alpha-tocopherol or DL-alpha-tocopherol is vitamin E's naturally occurring form. Vitamin E functions as an antioxidant, preventing damage to cell membranes. As a free radical scavenger, it protects all tissues of the body, including the skin.

When applied directly to the skin, vitamin E penetrates the epidermis. It also reduces water loss through the skin and therefore protects against dryness.

Many people apply vitamin E to the skin in the hope that it will speed up healing. Experts tell us, though, that its ability to heal wounds from surgery or other types of skin trauma is unproved. Furthermore, topical application of vitamin E has a well-documented history of causing skin irritation. It is not recommended for people with Environmentally Sensitive Skin.

Researchers recently found that, taken orally, 1,000 IU of natural vitamin E plus 2,000 milligrams of vitamin C boosted resistance to sunburn by 20 percent. These studies are preliminary, and you should not consider vitamin E to be photoprotective.

As an oral supplement, it is recommended that you take 200 to 400 IU daily.

To use after sun exposure, buy in capsule form, break open the capsules and apply.

■ ■

Warning

People scheduled for surgery should not take vitamin E because it promotes bleeding and bruising.

■ ■

Dietary sources of vitamin E are sunflower seeds, walnuts, almonds and wheat germ oil.

VITAMIN C

Another important antioxidant for healthy skin is vitamin C (ascorbic acid). Oral vitamin C promotes wound healing and is essential for the synthesis of collagen.

Like vitamin E, vitamin C protects the skin from damage produced by ultraviolet light. In the process of protecting your skin, two-thirds of the skin's natural vitamin C is destroyed and thus needs to be replenished. Although vitamin C does not function as a sunscreen, it appears to provide some protection against adverse reactions to the sun. It should not be used as a sunscreen, however.

Sailors deprived of vitamin C on long voyages developed a condition called scurvy. A British naval surgeon found that citrus rapidly cured scurvy. Even in modern times, scurvy exists among persons who are deprived of adequate vitamin C, such as the institutionalized elderly, the poor and alcoholics. Signs of scurvy include coiled hairs on the body with bleeding in the follicles, gingivitis and poor wound healing.

While only 10 milligrams of ascorbic acid are needed to fend off scurvy, researchers have engaged in elaborate studies to determine whether larger doses can provide additional benefits to the human body, including the skin. The current recommended daily allowance in the United States is 60 milligrams. Many researchers believe even this recommendation is too low, especially for those who smoke and for women who are pregnant or breastfeeding.

In one report, researchers suggested that vitamin C may play an important role for skin care in three different situations:

Wound healing. Vitamin C supplements offer benefits for healing wounds. Studies show that postsurgical wounds heal abnormally more frequently in persons with low levels of ascorbic acid.

Aging skin. When ascorbic acid is added to skin components in the laboratory, growth is stimulated. Thus, researchers reason that supplemental vitamin C may slow skin aging.

Prevention of skin cancer. In animal studies, dietary ascorbic acid has been shown to delay the incidence of skin tumors induced by ultraviolet radiation.

Vitamin C–based lotions, if properly formulated, may be an important aid in better-looking skin. An effective vitamin C–based cream has long been a quest in the cosmetics market. Delivering this vitamin to the skin presents a perplexing problem for several reasons.

Two characteristics are critical for a vitamin-based cream to do any good. It must penetrate the skin and remain potent after being exposed to the air. In the past, vitamin C could not be used topically because it could not fulfill either requirement. New technological advances may provide the necessary penetration and potency needed.

In order for a vitamin C cream to have a noticeable effect on your skin, the vitamin must be present in concentrations of more than 10 percent. A careful study has demonstrated that a formulation of 10 percent ascorbic acid results in a more rapid resolution of redness after laser surgery of the skin. Topical vitamin C may play an important role in the prevention and treatment of other skin inflammations as well.

If the cream or lotion can penetrate the skin and remain potent, the vitamins within the product may prevent certain types of UVA and UVB radiation damage and have anti-inflammatory effects.

Warning

High concentrations of vitamin C can cause irritations such as redness and stinging.

As an oral supplement, it is recommended that you take 500 to 1,500 milligrams daily. Use vitamin C–based creams if you find Retin-A and/or alpha hydroxy acid products too irritating. Vitamin C products should be used within thirty to ninety days after opening. Your best bet is to store the cream in the refrigerator and discard it if it turns dark brown or smells rancid.

Recommended products are AVON ANEW FORMULA C FACIAL TREATMENT CAPSULES and CELLEX-C SKIN-FIRMING CREAM.

Dietary sources of vitamin C are sweet peppers and bell peppers, oranges, grapefruit, collard greens and kiwi.

Soothing Herbs

Treating diseases with herbs is neither new nor limited to alternative medicine practitioners. One-quarter of the drugs we use today are either plant-derived or synthesized versions of plant compounds. Traditional practitioners still employ one of the earliest and best-known herbs, foxglove (digitalis), to treat heart disease. Willow bark yielded the main ingredient in aspirin, and snakeroot was the source for reserpine (a diuretic).

The cosmetic industry is always on the lookout for safe and effective natural products because of the built-in consumer appeal. Many herbal remedies derive from folklore and testimonials, so I am always interested in finding a scientific study of herbs and their effect on the skin. One such study was conducted in which six herbs were tested for efficacy. The results were quite impressive. Below is a list of the herbs and a description of their potential usefulness:

Yucca glauca, also known as Mojave yucca or soapweed. Used traditionally to treat burns and abrasions. Yucca glauca was demonstrated to reduce skin irritation by about 75 percent compared to treatment with a placebo.

Meadowsweet, also known as Filipendula rubra, queen of the prairie, dolloff and bridewort. Used traditionally to treat burns and abrasions. This herb is recognized as a type of natural aspirin.

Wild geranium (Geranium maculatum). Used traditionally to treat canker sores, sunburn and inflammation. The scientific study evaluated this herb for its effect on skin smoothness. After six weeks of use, there was a significant reduction in wrinkles and an increase in hydration of the skin.

Hawthorn, also known as Maybloom and Whitehorn. Used traditionally to reduce inflammation and to improve circulation. The study evaluated this herb for its effect on acne. After four weeks of treatment, acne was reduced by 35 percent as compared to a control group, and a 69 percent reduction in bacteria was observed.

Garden balsam reduced sunburn redness.

Clintonia borealis also reduced sunburn and increased cell growth.

Although the research is preliminary, the above herbs do show promise as a new approach to skin care.

Herb Preparation Terms

Poultice: Moistened chopped herbs held in place with a bandage that is applied directly to the skin.

Compress: Clean cloths dipped in an herbal solution. I recommend thin cloth diapers that have been washed several times.

Infusion: Similar to the way one makes tea except the herbs are left in the hot water to steep for ten to twenty minutes.

Decoction: Tea made from root herbs. Place herbs in water, bring to a boil, then simmer for ten to twenty minutes.

Tincture: Steeping herbs in drinkable alcohol, such as vodka. Use from 40 proof to almost 200 proof.

Essential Oils: How They Work and How to Use Them

Essential oils, the distilled extracts from plants, have been used for at least five thousand years. The flowers, leaves, roots, seeds and even skins of plants are used to create essential oils. The oils are what give plants and flowers their fragrances. Hormones, vitamins and other natural elements are found in essential oils. In their natural form, essential oils vary in concentration. Synthetic oils, by contrast, are man-made but have a more consistent composition. Experts tell us that synthetic and natural essential oils work equally well.

No one knows exactly how essential oils work. We do know, however, that essential oils are absorbed through the skin into the bloodstream. The eyelids, behind the ears and inside the wrist provide the easiest access because the skin is thinnest in those areas. (See warnings on use on pages 259 to 260.) By contrast, the soles, palms, forehead, scalp and underarms tend to have thicker, less penetrable skin.

The best essential oils for your Skin Profile are as follows:

Hormonally or Stress Reactive: lavender, geranium, ylang-ylang, jasmine.

Environmentally Sensitive: chamomile, rose. (Always use essential oil in low dilution for Environmentally Sensitive Skin—1 percent or less.) Use only one type of oil at a time in order to rule out allergic reactions.

Overexposed or Hearty: geranium, neroli, frankincense.

Joni Loughran, in "Aromatherapy for Skin and Hair Care," recommends these simple strategies for essential skin care:

● Drop eight to ten drops of essential oil for your Skin Profile in the bath. Use warm water to relax or cool water to invigorate or calm inflammation.

● Massage your body with essential oil. Add twenty to twenty-five drops of essential oil to two ounces of canola or other vegetable oil. If your skin tends to break out, rinse with a mild soap-and-water shower after the massage.

● Make a facial compress: Add two to five drops of essential oil to a basin filled with water, stir, then immerse a clean washcloth. Squeeze out excess water and apply cloth to face.

● Add essential oil to simple moisturizing products, ten to twenty drops for every two ounces.

NATURAL REMEDIES FOR IRRITATIONS AND INFLAMMATIONS

Calendula cream, also known as Golden Marigold, has long been touted as useful in reducing inflammation. It is used in Germany for the reduction of inflammation and to promote healing. Calendula is also widely accepted as a topical treatment for diaper rash. According to James Duke in *The Green Pharmacy,* calendula stimulates the production of white blood cells that help to fight harmful microbes. He recommends purchasing calendula flower ointment and applying as necessary.

How to use: Pour one cup of boiling water over one to two teaspoons of the herb and allow to steep for ten minutes. Can be used as a gargle or mouthwash for mouth sores. Pour brewed tea into a clean, absorbent cloth and apply to irritated skin after the tea has sufficiently cooled. You can also purchase calendula cream in health food stores.

Chamomile contains anti-inflammatory agents that can quiet irritations and soothe sensitive areas. The most studied type of chamomile is known as "pure" or "German" chamomile. The plant oils in chamomile have been proven by scientific investigation to contain such fatty acids as azulene, which is essential to human health. Chamomile may also be useful in healing sunburn, eczema and psoriasis. In one German study, chamomile was found to have an effect that was 60 percent as active as .25% hydrocortisone when applied topically.

Although chamomile is considered extremely safe, certain persons with allergies to grass and ragweed may develop an allergic reaction.

How to use: Put a handful of dried chamomile flowers into a bowl. Slowly pour boiling water over the flowers, stirring until they make a mush. Allow to cool. Wrap in a clean, soft cloth and apply. Leave on for fifteen minutes.

Cucumber is a soother for dermatitis and, some even say, smooths wrinkles.

How to use: Puree in a blender and leave on the affected area for fifteen minutes to one hour.

Wild Pansy eases itching from eczema and soothes acne.

How to use: Steep one teaspoon of herb per cup of tea for ten minutes. Let cool, then apply directly.

Saint-John's-Wort has received the most attention lately for its antidepressant effects, but it is also valued for its healing and antibacterial properties in the treatment of bruises, burns and cuts.

How to use: Apply directly to the wound. May be purchased as an infused oil.

Lavender, the lovely scented flower, soothes cuts, sunburns and insect bites.

How to use: Prepare your bath with Epsom salts, colloidal oatmeal (AVEENO BATH) and lavender oil. Soak in the tub for fifteen minutes. Never use more than seven drops of lavender oil in the tub.

Jewelweed may reduce irritation from poison ivy, poison oak and poison sumac. I have previously discussed traditional and home remedies for poison ivy. Herbalists claim that jewelweed, used internally or externally, can provide relief.

How to use: Mash fresh leaves and apply over rash.

Witch Hazel is a powerful astringent and works about as well as 1 percent hydrocortisone to relieve itching and minor skin inflammations. Great for soothing sunburns. *Do not confuse this herb with commercial witch hazel liquid.* Distilled witch hazel, available over the counter in the United States, is totally devoid of an ingredient called tannins, thought to be of use in the treatment of dermatitis. It is best to prepare fresh witch hazel leaves as directed below.

How to use: Simmer one ounce of witch hazel bark and one pint of water for ten minutes. Strain and allow to cool. Dip a clean cotton cloth in the mixture, wring and apply for thirty minutes. To soothe irritated patches of eczema, bathe with an infusion of herbal witch hazel diluted in warm water.

Parsley. To reduce the appearance of black-and-blue marks, keep a "parsley ice cube" handy. Chop parsley, mix with warm water and then freeze the mixture in an ice cube tray. At the first sign of a bruise, apply the cube to the skin. Be sure the skin is not cut or open. Try a cube under each eye as well to reduce the appearance of dark circles.

Arnica oil is very useful for bruises. It can be applied directly to the injured area. Homeopathic arnica 30X can be taken internally to help bruises heal faster.

Aloe vera. Almost everyone knows about the benefits of aloe vera for burns, sunburn and other minor skin irritations as well as wound healing. It has antifungal, antibacterial and anti-inflammatory properties. It contains many compounds, such as vitamins C and E and zinc, which are necessary for wound healing. It also contains folic acid.

Studies have shown it to be as effective as a topical drug called silvadine, which is commonly used by doctors for the treatment of first- and second-degree burns. Therefore, it can be applied directly to minor burns.

Active compounds in aloe have a tendency to decompose quickly, which compromises effectiveness. There has been little success in stabilizing aloe. In addition, most aloe-based products do not list the percentage of aloe present. A concentration of at least 70 percent is needed for aloe to produce antimicrobial benefits, but in most aloe-based products there is not nearly enough to do any good at all.

Fresh aloe gel has been shown to promote the attachment and

growth of cells, but commercial products containing aloe gel can be toxic and harmful to skin. Experts tell us that the only way to assure aloe's effects is to use fresh gel from the plant. Keep one in your home, and when needed, cut off a piece of the leaf and apply the gel directly to your skin. A natural recipe for using aloe vera leaves is as follows: Wash the leaves. Cut each piece in half to expose the largest amount of gel. Wrap each piece in plastic and date it. When you need the leaves, remove the plastic and apply the side of the leaf to the skin. Smear the gel over the affected area or hold in place with a bandage.

HERPES SIMPLEX

In chapter 13 I discussed the traditional medical treatments for cold sores and fever blisters, also known as herpes simplex. If, however, you want to try an herbal remedy, MELISSA BALM is recommended. In Europe a concentrated extract of Melissa that is marketed for the treatment of both oral and genital herpes is said to shorten healing time. You can make your own solution in the United States by preparing a strong tea from two to three teaspoons of finely cut leaves and one-half cup of water. Apply to the lesion with a cotton ball several times a day. There have been no significant side effects reported.

Another remedy is Lemon Balm Extract 1% cream. In a 1996 study, healing time was significantly shorter in the group using the balm than in the placebo group.

■ Calming Acne Naturally

The standard medical therapies for acne include topical and systemic antibiotics as well as Retin-A and related medications, including Accutane. All of these therapies have side effects. I generally prescribe Accutane only to the person who has been suffering with cystic acne and has had no response to other therapies. Many men and women, however, with milder forms of acne still want effective therapy without side effects.

Tea Tree Oil. One of the best studied herbal treatments for acne is tea tree oil. It kills the bacteria which cause acne and works as an all-around first-aid treatment and antiseptic for speeding skin healing. Naturopaths tell us that tea tree oil is an ideal skin disinfectant and is effective against strains of organisms that cause acne.

How to use: Tea tree oil should be applied to acne or irritated skin in a diluted form, usually one part tea tree oil to 10 parts spring water in the evening. Apply with a cotton ball after a gentle washing with water. It is best to make a fresh "batch" of tea tree lotion each time you wash. Oral ingestion of tea tree oil is not recommended as this could lead to a toxic reaction.

A recommended tea tree oil product is RACHEL PERRY PERFECTLY CLEAR HERBAL ANTISEPTIC.

Azelaic Acid. It is now found in a prescription-strength retinoid cream called AZELEX, which has been proven to treat acne. The basic ingredient can be purchased over the counter, however, and should be prepared in a 20 percent solution.

Vitamins. Recommended herbal treatments for acne include the following: 10,000 IU per day of vitamin A; 400 IU per day of vitamin E; and 30 milligrams per day of zinc (zinc gluconate or zinc picolinate).

Warning

Herbs and vitamins need to be used for weeks to months for optimal results.

Herbal Recommendations for Eczema, Psoriasis, Dermatitis

Throughout this chapter, I will be discussing alternative treatments for conditions such as eczema, psoriasis and other chronic conditions.

The treatment of choice for these skin problems by the traditional medical community has been steroids, either in cream or pill form.

When steroids were first discovered, the medical community thus hailed them as a miracle cure for a host of disorders. As the years passed, we began to understand that steroids had potent side effects.

Steroids work by limiting the immune response and thus reducing inflammation. They actually shut down the body's internal reactions that cause skin eruptions. Steroids are available in pill, cream, lotion and ointments, both over the counter and by prescription. Long-term use of steroid cream can cause atrophy of the skin, which looks thinned, shiny and wrinkled. This can even occur with over-the-counter–strength products.

Steroids in pill form are generally stronger than topical products and affect the whole body. Side effects of long-term steroid use include osteoporosis, cataracts, glaucoma, high blood pressure, weight gain, stomach ulcers and susceptibility to infections.

Someone who is itchy, irritated and embarrassed by eczema wants fast and complete relief, and in those cases, when appropriate, I do prescribe steroids. For the person who wants to try a more natural approach, however, patience promises great rewards.

Many of my patients with irritated skin such as eczema, psoriasis and dermatitis have told me that they have achieved positive results by using two capsules three times daily of Evening Primrose Oil. Evening Primrose Oil contains gamma linolenic acid (GLA). In Great Britain, GLA is an approved product for the treatment of eczema.

PSORIASIS

Evening Primrose is best used in conjunction with steroid creams and exposure to ultraviolet radiation for serious cases of psoriasis. For example, I ask patients who are interested in utilizing herbal remedies to use steroid creams for three days, then Evening Primrose Oil for one day. If there is an improvement, I suggest that they use prescription medicine at night and Evening Primrose Oil during the day because it has a much more pleasant odor. With a certain amount of experimentation with alternate treatments, patients may be able to reduce the frequency or strength of steroids.

Taking Evening Primrose Oil capsules (3,000 milligrams daily) is also recommended. Very few side effects have been reported.

Omega-3 and Omega-6 fatty acids are known as essential fatty acids. Our bodies do not make EFAs, and we must get them from our diet. They are a very important precursor to a group of compounds called eicosanoids which, among other functions, act as anti-inflammatories. Since many chronic skin conditions have an underlying inflammatory component and since most people do not have adequate EFA's in their diet, supplements can be very useful. Omega-6 is easy to get in our diet. It is contained in soybean oil, safflower oil, sunflower oil and sesame oil. By contrast, omega-3 is a bit harder to get in the diet for most people. Salmon, flaxseeds and rapeseed are good sources. Both omega-3 and omega-6 can be taken as a supplement in the form of Evening Primrose Oil capsules as recommended above.

Andrew Weil, M.D., the well-known author of *Spontaneous Healing,* suggests eliminating milk and milk products from your diet to treat atopic dermatitis. Try drinking soy or rice milk for a week or two. The flavor may take some getting used to, but it is worth it—especially considering the good news we hear about soy instead of cow's milk in the prevention of cancer. For an herbal remedy to treat atopic dermatitis, Dr. Weil suggests 500 milligrams of black currant oil twice a day taken orally, plus the application of aloe vera gel and calendula lotion or cream. He also says that chaparral tea used topically can soothe irritated skin.

Perhaps the best plant-derived product for psoriasis is capsaicin, the principal ingredient in cayenne pepper. One study found that the application of capsaicin cream led to a significant reduction in scaling and erythema (redness) over a six-week period. In another study, patients with psoriasis found that scaling, thickness, erythema and itching were substantially reduced over the six weeks.

ECZEMA
Dietary: Evening primrose oil or flaxseed oil, two capsules, three times a day. Zinc gluconate or zinc picolinate, 30 milligrams per day. Take a B-complex supplement every day and make sure that the tablet contains good levels of niacin (B_3).

Topical: Apply calendula and comfrey cream or salve, two to three times a day. (Eclectic Institute makes a calendula-comfrey cream that is very nice.)

Blackberry leaf tea can be used topically.

Aloe vera gel from the leaf of the plant will encourage healing. Apply licorice or licorice extract cream two times per day.

Herbs: Drink burdock root and nettle tea. Use dry bulk herbs if possible. Place approximately one rounded teaspoon of the herbs in a cup or teapot, pour one cup of boiling water on top, and steep for thirty to sixty minutes, covered for best effect. May be sweetened or flavored with honey or your favorite tea if desired. Drink three cups per day. (Tea can be made in quantities for up to three days at a time and stored in the refrigerator.)

Other anti-inflammatory herbs that may help to heal eczema include chamomile and red clover.

Black currant oil can be used on the skin, and 500 milligrams of black currant oil tablets twice a day can be taken for allergic dermatitis.

Chinese Herbal Therapy for Dermatitis

Traditional Chinese medicine, a four-thousand-year-old science, seeks to treat the whole person rather than the individual disease. It's difficult to argue with that approach. Therapy is based on the interpretation of signs and symptoms encompassing the philosophy of yin and yang. In a healthy body, yin and yang are in perfect balance. Another fundamental concept in Chinese medicine is qi. This has been translated as "energy," "material force" and "vital power." Skin disease is perceived as a breakdown in the relationship between the yin nourishment and yang activity—in other words, the result of internal disharmony.

In a well-prepared clinical trial, Chinese herbs were given to people with uninfected atopic dermatitis. The patients in the study continued with their steroid creams and lotions. The Chinese herbal treatment, originally formulated in the year 1119, contained *Ledebouriella seseloides, P. chinensis, Akebai clematidis, R. glutinosa, Paeonia latiflora, L. gracile, Dictamnus dasycarpus, Tribulus terrestris, G. glabrae* and *S. tenuifolia.*

In the study, patients who used both steroids and the Chinese herbs showed rapid and continued improvement in their conditions; both the amount and intensity of their skin irritation diminished. Further studies showed that Chinese herbal therapy produced a sustained remission of disease activity in patients with atopic skin disorders who had been unresponsive to a variety of conventional treatments.

Licorice root is also commonly used in traditional Chinese herbal medicine for atopic dermatitis. A traditional formulation of ten herbs including licorice root has been widely studied in Great Britain for atopic dermatitis. The combination has proven successful in the long-term study of children and the short-term study of adults.

Warnings About Treating Atopic Dermatitis Herbally

If you have had very little relief despite traditional treatments, you may want to consider alternative methods for your chronic atopic dermatitis. Before you do this, however, I recommend the following guidelines:

1 Do not use herbal or any alternative therapies until you have seen a dermatologist who can diagnose your condition. Other, more serious conditions can mimic dermatitis.

2 Do not use herbal or alternative therapies if your skin is infected or oozing.

3 Inform your dermatologist of your intention to try herbal medicine so that he or she may determine if you have any medical conditions that may preclude its safe use. For example, people taking Accutane should never take vitamin A.

4 Continue to use topical treatments per your doctor's recommendation.

5 Be certain that the alternative practitioner you are dealing with has the correct credentials. Get references from friends and other patients.

6 If you experience any side effects, such as a headache, dizziness, drowsiness or a worsening of your skin condition, see your doctor and discontinue the herbal therapy.

Nasty Naturals

Having praised natural substances, I must inject a warning. Because many of these products are unregulated, it is sometimes difficult to guarantee purity and ensure reproducible, standardized finished products. Many types of essential oils are known skin irritants. These include cassia, cinnamon bark, cinnamon leaf, cumin, lemongrass, oregano, clove stem, clove bud, wild or creeping thyme and red thyme.

Other essential oils may render the skin hypersensitive to ultraviolet rays. Avoid these oils if you have sensitive skin: angelica root, lime, bitter orange, bergamot, lemon, cumin, lovage, fig leaf, savin and verbena.

Warning

Keep these admonitions in mind when using essential oils:

1 Essential oils must be diluted. Always check with a reliable herbalist regarding how to dilute them.
2 Excessive or inappropriate use of essential oils can lead to headaches, nausea, even death.
3 A limited range of essential oils should be used to cover the specific requirements of the condition being treated.

BEWARE THE HERBAL HYPE

If you are considering taking the herbal path to beauty, keep alert. A responsible person, however enthusiastic about herbal treatments, will acknowledge that some herbs are dangerous. Herbs are considered "foods" rather than drugs by the FDA. Because of this, they need not come with warnings or directions as do other over-the-counter products.

Be skeptical when you hear any of these claims. All of these statements are *false:*

1 The medical establishment is leading a conspiracy against the use of herbs.

2 Herbs cannot harm, only cure.

3 Whole herbs are more effective than their isolated active constituents.

4 "Natural" and "organic" herbs are superior to synthetic drugs. (In fact, the opposite may be true.)

5 Reducing the dose of medicine increases its therapeutic value. (This is often claimed by practitioners of homeopathic treatment.)

6 Physiological tests in animals are not applicable to human beings. (Groundbreaking and effective treatments on humans often have their origins with their use in animals.)

7 Anecdotal evidence is highly significant.

The information in this chapter can be used to approach natural healing in a balanced and informed manner. For those of you who are ardent supporters of natural healing, my suggestions may sound a bit conservative, but my approach has always been that of a skeptical scientist with an open mind. Using herbs and other natural modalities safely requires care and prudence. One of my favorite things about using herbs is the self-empowerment it provides to those patients who have hit a brick wall with the use of traditional medicine in the treatment of their skin condition. My second favorite aspect of natural healing is how it causes some of us to take a second look at the way we approach our body's tremendous ability to heal from within.

15

Twenty-First-Century Skin Care

Safe tans, bloodless plastic surgery, genetically engineered perfect skin. Are these the new cosmetic techniques for the next century? It's foolish to rule anything out. Who would have imagined all the advances that this century has already brought us—from antibiotics to laser surgery. I often think that my young daughter will find our late-twentieth-century beauty methods charmingly antiquated, if not barbaric—face-lifts, acids, hair transplants. These treatments may sound as quaint to her as a nonportable telephone sounds to you.

Many of the most innovative and practical advances to be made in dermatology will depend on the answer to one important question: How does normal skin behave? It seems like a simple question (so many important questions are), but its answer will give us the methods to correct skin that is abnormal—sun-damaged, itchy, vulnerable.

I am looking forward to practicing medicine in the coming century. My patients will be beneficiaries of innovations in technology and medicine.

The practice of dermatology will shift from the scalpel to the pill. We will, I believe, uncover treatments for skin disorders that will reduce the need for surgery. For example, when we finally discover what causes male baldness, hair transplants will become obsolete. Instead, we will develop medicine that will stimulate hair growth in specific areas of the body. Better yet, we will intercede and stop hair loss before it occurs. Many people who use current products for hair loss are disappointed with the results or bothered by the side effects. New technology will provide people with a simple test that can predict whether a particular type of drug will work to grow hair.

With respect to skin cancer, our efforts to defeat this sometimes deadly disease may come from vaccines. Several of these vaccines are in development for patients who already have melanoma. Newer vaccines may someday be used for high-risk individuals in an effort to prevent the cancer from developing. Our methods of cancer detection will grow increasingly sophisticated and specific. It will not be long before we will be able to detect cancer by the presence of a single cell within our body.

Retinoids, the best known of which is Retin-A, were introduced fifteen years ago. In that short amount of time, they have dramatically changed the way dermatologists treat acne and aging skin. Retinoids affect cell growth and sebaceous gland activity. Seizing on this important mechanism, scientists are now refining retinoids for exciting new uses. Retinoids are now used experimentally to treat a type of leukemia. The development of receptor-specific retinoids for the topical treatment of psoriasis, acne and other skin disorders may lead to other effective new compounds. In other words, diseases like psoriasis may be cured instead of just treated. Retinoids may also reverse skin cancer and disorders of skin pigmentation.

Like retinoids, antiviral drugs arrived on the medical scene only in the last decade, but in that short amount of time they have improved the quality of life and life span for many people. Today we can only suppress viruses. Tomorrow we may cure them with more potent and specific antiviral drugs. Cells infected with viruses will be targeted by drugs while healthy cells are spared, thereby reducing side effects. Our greatest triumph in the use of antivirals will be the development of a drug that can conquer HIV.

Vaccination therapy against viruses and other diseases is also being developed. The success of the polio and smallpox vaccines demonstrates that prevention needs to be our goal.

A better collagen. Smoothing out lines, wrinkles and scars with collagen is a far-from-perfect procedure. For one thing, collagen lasts only a few months because it degrades and is absorbed into the body. Another problem is that some people are allergic to collagen.

The FDA is now reviewing for approval a special material called polymethyl methacrylate (PMMA) that can be used with collagen for better results. In essence, PMMA can be considered a collagen quilt, surrounding the collagen. PMMA is now used in Europe, South America, Canada and a number of other countries. The three attributes of PMMA—smooth, biodegradable and inert—make it a much better material for injection into the skin than collagen alone. PMMA actually consists of microscopic beads that cause the surrounding human tissue to create natural fibrous material. After being injected, the beads are immediately encapsulated into a patient's own collagen fibers, holding the collagen in place and even allowing for easy removal if necessary.

Another development in the area of "fillers" for lines and scars on the skin is a material called Hyaluron or Hyalin gel. Although it is not yet approved by the FDA, it has been on the market in Europe for some years. It is a constituent of ground substance, the naturally occurring "cement" that holds our skin together, rather than a collagen material. Finally, scientists are developing a technology that will actually "turn on" our skin's collagen formation to develop what is needed to look younger.

A better sunscreen. We have made a lot of progress in developing highly protective types of sunscreen, but no sunscreen guards against all harmful ultraviolet radiation. Researchers are working on a product that contains synthetic melanin. It is supposed to provide better protection because it absorbs rather than deflects dangerous rays. This discovery may not only lead to a safe way to tan but it also may increase the skin's resistance to ultraviolet damage. In the coming century we may witness the development of techniques that will prevent all photoaging of the skin. This may be in the form of a systemic sunscreen that blocks harmful ultraviolet radiation better than any cream or lotion.

Gene therapy. We will be able to identify people who are predisposed to certain diseases through genetic research, and we will be able to intervene before the disease even manifests itself. By using drugs comprised of DNA fragments, we will also be able to treat diseases after they appear. The skin is an especially promising target for gene therapy because is it readily available for repeated administration of a drug and is easy to monitor. Researchers are particularly enthusiastic about treating eczema and allergic skin reactions with gene therapy.

Enhanced delivery systems. Drugs and active ingredients will become more potent as we develop ways to deliver them more efficiently through the skin. Researchers are working on substances that can enhance skin penetration. Estrogen, nicotine (to aid in quitting smoking) and pain medication are already delivered through skin patches. I expect that other drugs and treatments will be administered this way, enhancing the quality of life for many.

My goal when writing this book has been to provide you with the tools and information that you need to feel good about the way you look. It has been my experience time and time again that when people learn how to care for their skin, wonderful things start to happen. The author Anne Lamott has written extensively about her struggles with eating disorders and issues of self-esteem tied to her appearance. Anyone familiar with her work can see that she is deeply spiritual, sensitive and insightful. I was moved by a passage in her most recent book, *Traveling Mercies,* in which she explains why it is necessary to pay attention to the way one looks. She writes, "Sometimes you start with the outside and get it right. You tend to your spirit through your body. It's polishing the healthy young skin of that girl who was here just a moment ago and who still lives inside." Caring about how we look to the outside world communicates a sense of self value, worth and respect. We don't need to apologize for wanting to look good.

Looking attractive, healthy and youthful (though not necessarily young) has always provided its possessors with an advantage. The problems start when we focus on our appearance at the expense of developing other important personal qualities.

No single medical innovation in the field of cosmetic medicine will ever erase all signs of aging and other unwanted skin problems. And perhaps that's a good thing. It's good because daily beauty rituals from washing our face to clipping our nails keep us in touch with our bodies and force us to spend time with ourselves. They are really not mundane tasks when considered in that perspective. Many of us spend a lot of time caring for others—children, spouses, parents, friends. At the end of the day, we are exhausted. Taking care of our skin "forces" us to take time to attend to our own needs.

Developing a relationship with your skin helps you to keep in touch with other aspects of your well-being. With this book, I hope to introduce you to the subtle and not so subtle signs that your skin gives you when it needs attention. It is intended to help you realize that by paying attention to your skin, its changing nature, its delicate composition, you will also be caring for your inner self.

Bibliography

"A Primer on Cosmetics." American Academy of Dermatology, 1991.

Alster and West. "Effect of Topical Vitamin C on Postoperative Carbon Dioxide Laser Resurfacing Erythema." *Dermatologic Surgery* 24 (1998): 331–34.

Baker, Thomas J., M.D., guest ed. "Skin Resurfacing." *Clinics in Plastic Surgery.* Philadelphia: W. B. Saunders Company, January 1998.

Begoun, Paula. *The Beauty Bible.* Seattle: Beginning Press, 1997.

Benson, Linda R. "Sun-Free Tanning May Be Possible Without Risk of UV Exposure." *Dermatology Times* 19, no. 2 (February 1998): 58–59.

Bernhard, Jeffrey D., M.D. *Itch: Mechanisms and Management of Pruritus.* New York: McGraw-Hill, 1994.

Blackmun, Susie. "Atopic Dermatitis: No Cure, But Carefully Selected Treatments Work." *Dermatology Times* 19, no. 8 (August 1998): 37.

Bridgett, Christopher, Peter Noren, and Richard Staughton. *Atopic Skin Disease.* Petersfield, UK: Wrightson Biomedical Publishing, Ltd., 1996.

Brinton, D. G., M.D., and George Napheys, M.D. *The Laws of Health in Relation to the Human Form.* Springfield: W. J. Holland, 1870.

Brody, Jane E. "Restoring Ebbing Hormones May Slow Aging." *The New York Times,* July 18, 1995.

Brown, Donald J., N.D., and Alan M. Dattner. "Phytotherapeutic Approaches to Common Dermatologic Conditions." *Archives of Dermatology* 134 (1998): 1401–1404.

Carper, Jean. *Stop Aging Now!* New York: HarperCollins, 1995.

Colven, Roy M., and Sheldon R. Pinnell. "Topical Vitamin C in Aging." *Clinics in Dermatology* 14 (1996): 227–34.

Connolly, John J., Ed. D. *How to Find the Best Doctors.* 3d ed. New York: Castle Connolly Medical Ltd., 1998.

Darr, Douglas, et al. "Effectiveness of Antioxidants (Vitamin C and E) With and Without Sunscreens as Topical Photoprotectants." *Acta Derm Venereol (Stockh)* 76 (1996): 264–68.

De Botton, Alain. *How Proust Can Change Your Life.* New York: Pantheon Books, 1997.

DeGroot, Anton C., M.D., Ph.D. "Fatal Attractiveness: The Shady Side of Cosmetics." *Clinics in Dermatology* 16 (1998): 167–79.

Denerstein, Lorraine, and Julia Shelley, eds. *A Woman's Guide to Menopause and Hormone Replacement Therapy.* Washington, DC: American Psychiatric Press, Inc., 1998.

Denham, Harman. "Role of Antioxidant Nutrients in Aging: Overview." *Age* 18 (April 1995): 2–5.

Draelos, Zoe Diana, M.D. "Skin Facts." New York University School of Medicine, Winter 1998.

Draelos, Zoe Diana, M.D. *Cosmetics in Dermatology,* 2d edition. New York: Churchill Livingstone, 1995.

Draelos, Zoe Diana, M.D. "Basic Tenets in the Evaluation of Cosmetics and Skin Care Products." *The Journal of Clinical Dermatology* (Winter 1998): 35.

Draelos, Zoe Diana, M.D. "New Developments in Cosmetics and Skin Care Products." *Advances in Dermatology* 12 (1997): 3–15.

Duke, James A., Ph.D., et al. *The Green Pharmacy.* Emmaus, PA: Rodale Press, 1997.

Elson, Melvin, L., M.D. "Soft Tissue Augmentation: Update 1997." *Cosmetic Dermatology* (Winter 1998): 25.

Ersek, Robert A., M.D., et al. "Noninvasive Mechanical Body Contouring: A Preliminary Clinical Outcome Study." *Aesthetic Plastic Surgery* (1997): 61–67.

Fisher, Gary J., et al. "Pathophysiology of Premature Skin Aging Induced by Ultraviolet Light." *New England Journal of Medicine* 337 (1997): 1419–28.

Fitzpatrick, Thomas B., M.D., et al. *Dermatology in General Medicine.* New York: McGraw-Hill, 1993.

Fodor, Peter Bela, M.D. "Endermologie (LPG): Does It Work?" *Aesthetic Plastic Surgery* 21 (1997): 68–70.

Fradin, Mark, M.D. "Mosquitoes and Mosquito Repellents: A Clinician's Guide." *Annals of Internal Medicine* 128, no. 11 (1998): 931–34.

Gaynor, Alan, M.D. *Everything You Ever Wanted to Know About Cosmetic Surgery But Couldn't Afford to Ask.* New York: Broadway Books, 1998.

Gilchrist, B. A. "A Review of Skin Ageing and Its Medical Therapy." *British Journal of Dermatology* 135 (1996): 867–75.

Glogau, R. G. "Aesthetic and Anatomic Analysis of the Aging Skin. "Seminars in Cutaneous Medicine and Surgery," 15 (1996): 134–38.

Gottlieb, Bill, ed. *New Choices in Natural Healing.* Emmaus, PA: Rodale Press, Inc., 1995.

Grossbart, Ted A., and Carl Sherman. *Skin Deep.* Santa Fe: Health Press, 1992.

Haas, Elson M., M.D. *Staying Healthy with Nutrition.* Berkeley: Celestial Arts, 1992.

Havlik, Robert J., M.D. "Vitamin E and Wound Healing." *Plastic and Reconstructive Surgery* (December 1997): 1901–1902.

Jones, Heidi Emmerling. "Are They Just Skin Deep?" *RDH* (1998): 38–44.

Kabat-Zinn, J. "Influence of a Mindfulness Meditation-Based Stress Reduction Intervention on Rates of Skin Clearing in Patients with Moderate to Severe Psoriasis Undergoing Phototherapy (UVB) and Photochemotherapy (PUVA)." *Psychosomatic Medicine* 60 (1998): 624–32.

Kinney, Brian M., M.D. "External Fatty Tissue Massage (The 'Endermologie' and 'Silhouette' Procedures)." *Plastic and Reconstructive Surgery* (1997): 1903–1904.

Klein, Alan D., and Neil Penneys. "Aloe Vera." *Journal of the American Academy of Dermatology* 18 (1998): 714–19.

Korting, H. C., et al. "The Influence of the Regular Use of a Soap or an Acidic Syndet Bar on Pre-Acne," *Infection* 23, no. 2 (1995): 89–93.

Lamberg, Lynne. " 'Treatment' Cosmetics: Hype or Help." *Journal of the American Medical Association* 2790, no. 20 (1998): 1595–99.

Lamott, Anne. *Traveling Mercies: Some Thoughts on Faith.* New York: Pantheon Books, 1999.

Lewis, Carol. "Clearing Up Cosmetic Confusion." *FDA Consumer* (May–June 1998): 7–11.

Loughran, Joni. "Aromatherapy for Skin and Hair Care." *Energy Times* (March 1998): 54.

Memar, O. M., and S. K. Tyring. "Anti-Viral Agents in Dermatology, Current Status and Future Prospects." *International Journal of Dermatology,* vol. 34, no. 9 (1995): 597–606.

Mitchell, Deborah. "Daily Bathing Ameliorates Atopic Dermatitis in Young Children." *Dermatology Times* 19, no. 8 (1998): 43.

Murray Michael T., N.D. *The Healing Power of Herbs,* rvd. and expanded 2d ed. Rocklin: Prima Publishing, 1995.

Murray Michael T., N.D., et al. *Encyclopedia of Natural Medicine,* rvd. 2nd ed. Rocklin: Prima Publishing, 1997.

Perricone, Nicholas, M.D., ed. "Understanding the Use of Topical Anti-oxidants." *Skin and Aging* (January 1998): 18.

Peiss, Kathy Lee. *Hope in a Jar: The Making of America's Beauty Culture.* New York: Metropolitan Books, 1998.

Plewig, Gerd, and Albert M. Kligman. *Acne and Rosacea.* Berlin, Germany: Springer-Verlag, 1993.

Poucher, W. A. *Perfumes, Cosmetics and Soaps,* vol. 3, 9th ed. Norwell, MA: Chapman & Hall, 1993.

Price, Shirley, and Len Price. *Aromatherapy for Health Professionals.* Edinburgh: Churchill Livingstone, 1995.

Reiffel, Robert S., M.D. "Prevention of Hypertrophic Scars by Long-Term Paper Tape Application." *Plastic and Reconstructive Surgery* 96, no. 7 (1995): 1715–17.

Ringel, Eileen, M.D. "The Morality of Cosmetic Surgery for Aging." *Archives of Cosmetic Dermatology* (April 1998).

Scheinman, Pamela L. "Is It Really Fragrance-Free?" *American Journal of Contact Dermatitis* 8, no. 4 (1997): 239–42.

Scheman, Andrew J., M.D., and David L. Severson. *Pocket Guide to Medications Used in Dermatology,* 5th ed. Baltimore: Williams & Wilkins, 1997.

Schiavo, Mary, with Sabra Chartrand. *Flying Blind, Flying Safe.* New York: Avon Books, 1997.

Schoen, Linda Allen, M.D., and Paul Lazar. *The Look You Like.* New York: Marcel Dekker, Inc., 1990.

Scholz, D., and G. J. Brooks. "An Ethnobotanical Approach to the Development of Effective Cosmetic Actives." Abstract reprinted in International Business Communications, 2nd Annual International Industry Conference, Drug Discovery and Development Approaches to Cosmeceuticals, 1998.

Shealy, C. Norman, M.D., Ph.D. *The Illustrated Encyclopedia of Natural Remedies.* Boston: Element Books, 1998.

Sherris, David A., M.D., et al. "Management of Scar Contractures, Hypertrophic Scars and Keloids." *Otolaryngologic Clinics of North America* 28, no. 5 (1995): 1057–68.

Smith, Jeffrey B., M.D., and Neil A. Fenske. "Cutaneous Manifestations and Consequences of Smoking." *Journal of the American Academy of Dermatology* 34 (1996): 717–32.

Thompson, S. C. "Reduction of Solar Keratoses by Regular Sunscreen Use." *New England Journal of Medicine* 329 (1993): 1147–51.

Tyler, Varro E., Ph.D., Sc.D. *Herbs of Choice: The Therapeutic Use of Phytomedicinals.* New York: Pharmaceutical Products Press, 1994.

Uitto, Jouni, M.D., Ph.D. "Understanding Premature Skin Aging." *New England Journal of Medicine* 337 (1997): 1463–65.

Vail, Gilbert. *A History of Cosmetics in America.* New York: The Toilet Goods Association, Inc., 1947.

Warren, R. "The Influence of Hard Water (Calcium) and Surfactants on Irritant Contact Dermatitis." *Contact Dermatitis* 35 (1996): 337–43.

Warshaw, Erin. "Latex Allergy." *Journal of the American Academy of Dermatology* 39, no. 1 (1998).

Weil, Andrew, M.D. *Spontaneous Healing.* New York: Ballantine Books, 1996.

Weyers, Wolfgang, M.D. *Death of Medicine in Nazi Germany.* Philadelphia: Lippincott-Raven, 1998.

Winter, Ruth, M.S. *A Consumer's Dictionary of Cosmetic Ingredients,* 4th ed. New York: Three Rivers Press, 1994.

Wolf, Naomi. *The Beauty Myth.* New York: Anchor Books, 1992.

Wolf, R. "Entering the Twenty-First Century." *Clinics in Dermatology* (January–February 1996): 129–32.

Wolf, R. "Has Mildness Replaced Cleanliness Next to Godliness?" *Dermatology* 189 (1994): 217–21.

Wolfe, Sidney, M.D., et al. *10,289 Questionable Doctors.* Washington, DC: Public Citizen's Health Research Group, 1993.

Index

About the Authors

Dr. Barney Kenet is a leading authority on skin care in America. He is a dermatologic surgeon at New York Presbyterian Hospital/Cornell Medical Center and maintains a private practice in Manhattan. He is the founder and President of the American Melanoma Foundation and the coauthor of *Saving Your Skin: Prevention, Early Detection, and Treatment of Melanoma and Other Skin Cancers*. His wife, Patricia Lawler, is the coauthor of both books, a television producer and an attorney. They live in New York City with their daughter, Isabelle.